Acknowledgements

I would like to express my deep gratitude to all those who have contributed, directly or indirectly, to the development of this book. The power of minimalism is much more than a book; it's an inner journey, an invitation to lighten up our lives so that we can better savour what's essential.

Thank you to those close to me, for their constant support and patience, for giving me the space I needed to write, reflect and sometimes simply... do nothing. Your understanding was a real foundation.

I'd also like to thank all the readers who, through their sharing, their questions and their curiosity, fuel this movement towards a simpler, more aligned life. This book is addressed to you, and it is through you that it takes on its full meaning.

A special word for the thinkers, authors and artisans of minimalism who have inspired me throughout this journey: your words, your gestures and your commitment have ignited in me that spark which, today, I hope will enlighten others.

Finally, thank you to life, in all its complexity and beauty, which teaches us every day that true abundance often lies in the little when it is chosen with intention and love.

Claire Montel

CW01496999

Preamble

At a time when our lives are saturated with goods, information and constant demands, a silent aspiration is growing: that of a return to the essential. In a world that values quantity, speed and possession, minimalism is emerging not just as an aesthetic trend, but as a profound response to the excesses of our age.

The aim of this book, The power of minimalism, is not to convince you to live with three objects or to transform your home into a monochrome space. It proposes much more: a path of clarity, intention and freedom. It's for people who are feeling the weight of material, mental and relational clutter and who are looking for a more conscious, more aligned way of living.

In the first part, we explore what minimalism really is, overcoming clichés and misunderstandings. We'll see how this approach can lighten not only our spaces, but also our thoughts, our relationships and our habits. Then we'll get down to the nitty-gritty: how to apply minimalism to everyday life, from our homes to our screens, from our finances to our wardrobes. Finally, the last part will broaden the perspective: minimalism as a philosophy of life, as a tool for personal and spiritual transformation.

This book does not offer ready-made recipes, but an invitation to slow down, to question, to choose. It's not about depriving yourself, it's about freeing yourself. The power of minimalism lies in its ability to make room for ourselves, for others, for what really matters.

Contents

Introduction

Why minimalism?

At a time when everything seems to be moving ever faster, when notifications are invading our phones and advertising is relentlessly pushing us to consume, it's becoming essential to stop and ask ourselves a fundamental question: What if 'more' wasn't synonymous with 'better'? This is precisely where minimalism comes into its own. Much more than just a pared-down style or a bare white interior, minimalism is a philosophy of life, a conscious choice to free ourselves from the superfluous to make room for what really matters.

Free yourself from material clutter

Our society values accumulation. Having more objects, clothes and gadgets is often seen as a sign of success. Yet every object we own comes with an invisible burden: it takes up physical, mental and emotional space. We tidy, clean, maintain, insure, protect... and often feel overwhelmed.

Minimalism invites us to clear out the clutter, to keep only what is useful, beautiful or meaningful. By reducing the number of objects around us, we free up energy, time and clarity of mind. Fewer possessions mean less stress, fewer distractions and an easier time concentrating on what's essential.

Regain time and attention

Every useless object we own is a micro-distraction. Every superfluous activity we incorporate into our day distracts us from our real priorities. Minimalism isn't just about sorting out our cupboards: it extends to our timetable, our relationships and our commitments. It pushes us to say 'no' to what doesn't nourish us, in order to say a big 'yes' to what lifts us up.

In a world saturated with noise, minimalism acts like a filter. It helps us to be silent, to slow down, to become present to our lives again. It frees up time for deeply enriching activities: reading, meditating, creating, spending quality time with our loved ones, or simply doing nothing and enjoying the moment.

Refocus your life on what's essential

Minimalism is not deprivation. It's not about forcing yourself to live with the bare minimum in a spirit of sacrifice. On the contrary, it's a path towards a more meaningful life, where every object, every relationship, every activity is chosen with intention.

Adopting minimalism means doing some inner work: identifying what's really important to us, what corresponds to our deepest values, and sorting out the external noise from the inner voice. This takes courage. It requires us to free ourselves from social norms and the pressure of other people's opinions. But in return, it brings a kind of freedom that few other lifestyles can offer.

A positive impact on the planet

In a world faced with major ecological crises, minimalism is also a civic act. Reducing consumption, repairing instead of throwing things away, buying thoughtfully rather than impulsively - these are simple but powerful ways of preserving natural resources.

to preserve natural resources. By living with less, we are contributing to a more sustainable model of society, more respectful of the planet and future generations.

A response to the search for meaning

Many people today are looking to give meaning back to their lives. They feel an emptiness despite the professional success, possessions and distractions offered by consumer society. Minimalism is a response to this quest. By simplifying our lives, we can get to know ourselves better, clarify our aspirations and reconnect with what matters most: being, rather than having.

My journey towards a simpler life

Not so long ago, my life was like that of many people I meet today: cluttered, hectic, saturated with obligations and possessions. I was constantly chasing time, material possessions, success and the approval of others. Yet despite this frantic quest for 'more' - more objects, more comforts, more activities - I felt a persistent inner emptiness. An invisible weight was crushing me a little more every day. My physical space was overflowing with useless objects, just as my mind was overflowing with confused thoughts, anxieties and distractions.

Without realising it, I was living in a state of permanent overstimulation. My phone was ringing off the hook, notifications were flying, temptations to buy were everywhere, and I was saying 'yes' to everything for fear of missing out or disappointing someone. But by wanting to do everything, have everything, own everything, I'd forgotten myself.

I had forgotten myself. I no longer knew what really made me tick. I didn't know who I was, deep down.

Then, one day, I reached a breaking point. It wasn't a great tragedy, or a spectacular event. It was more like a discreet but powerful trigger, a profound weariness, a mental fatigue that I could no longer ignore. I looked around at my home, my relationships, my schedule, my mind and I saw chaos. I realised that this wasn't the life I wanted. I realised that I was living in excess, and that this excess was costing me my inner peace.

That's when I discovered minimalism. Not as a fad, nor as a cold aesthetic with white walls and Scandinavian furniture, but as a philosophy of life, a path towards the essential. I started small. A drawer emptied, a commitment declined, an application deleted. Each gesture gave me a breath of oxygen. The less I owned, the freer I felt. The less clutter I had, the more I found myself. I took the clutter out of my physical space, but also out of my thoughts, my relationships and my obligations. And what I discovered changed me profoundly.

Minimalism taught me to slow down, to choose with intention, to live with less in order to live better. It has allowed me to redefine my priorities, to create space for what really matters: inner peace, authentic relationships, health, creativity, the freedom to live according to my values.

This path towards a simpler life has not been linear. I've doubted, relapsed and hesitated. The modern world pushes us to consume and disperse ourselves, and going against the current takes courage. But at each stage, I felt a growing sense of calm. It's not a perfect destination, but a living process, a dynamic that I nurture every day with kindness.

Today, I may not have more money, a huge house or a luxury car. But I do have something far more precious: clarity, serenity and inner freedom. What I've gained in simplicity, I've regained in quality of life.

If you're reading this, it's probably because you too are feeling the call to something truer, calmer and more aligned. My hope in writing this book is to pass on to you the keys that have helped me to lighten up my life, so that you too can experience the power of minimalism.

Part I - Understanding Minimalism

Chapter 1: What is minimalism?

Modern and historical definitions

The modern definition of minimalism

In its modern conception, minimalism is much more than just a stripped-down aesthetic or a tendency to own fewer objects. It's a global philosophy of life, a deliberate choice to free ourselves from the superfluous in order to live a life aligned with our deepest values. It's not about restricting or depriving yourself, but about making room physically, mentally and emotionally for what really matters. In a world where abundance has become an often toxic norm, minimalism appears to be a lucid and powerful response to the overload of our times.

Modern minimalism is rooted in an awareness of compulsive accumulation. In our Western societies, success has long been associated with possession: the more you have, the better you're supposed to live. But this equation has proved misleading. Accumulating possessions, commitments, superficial relationships or digital distractions often ends up stifling what gives real meaning to life. Minimalism then becomes an act of gentle rebellion, a desire to break out of this consumerist spiral and rediscover what's essential: clarity, inner peace and freedom.

This way of life *is* based on a central question: "Does it bring me value? Every object, every activity, every relationship is filtered through this question. The aim is not to achieve an ideal number of possessions or to adhere to a rigid rule. Modern minimalism is personalised: it adapts to the needs, rhythms and sensibilities of each individual. For some, it means living in a small space with very few objects. For others, it may simply mean reducing their mental workload, simplifying their day, eliminating unnecessary noise and chaos.

In the material sphere, minimalism encourages us to free ourselves of non-essential possessions. Every object kept should have a concrete use or a strong emotional meaning. This process of decluttering is not about emptying your home to follow a fashion, but about creating a soothing, fluid and harmonious environment. An uncluttered space encourages clearer thinking, better sleep, reduced stress and even greater productivity. It's not just tidiness, it's a form of self-care.

In the digital world, minimalism takes on a new dimension. Our minds are constantly engaged by streams of information, notifications, social networks and advertising. Digital minimalism consists of taking back control of our attention, filtering what we consume, eliminating time-consuming applications and scheduling times to disconnect. This discipline allows us to reconnect with reality, preserve our mental health and, above all, rediscover quality time for ourselves, for others and for meaningful activities.

Minimalism also extends to human relationships. In a world where we often value the quantity of connections over their quality, this approach encourages us to sort things out. It encourages us to let go of toxic relationships, to reduce superficial interactions and to focus on deep, sincere, authentic relationships.

authenticity. This sorting out of relationships is not a rejection, but an act of loyalty to oneself. It allows us to nurture genuine relationships rather than dissipate ourselves in social appearances.

On a mental and emotional level, minimalism encourages a form of inner hygiene. It suggests simplifying thoughts, slowing down the frenetic pace imposed by modern society, and cultivating presence and full awareness. By letting go of unrealistic expectations, constant judgements and the race for performance, minimalism offers the possibility of fully inhabiting the moment, savouring what is, without always running towards what is missing. It's a practice o f refocusing, inner peace and stability.

Finally, financial minimalism is an essential pillar of this philosophy. It is based on the idea of spending with intention. This does not mean living in extreme frugality or denying yourself the pleasure of consumption, but rather learning to spend less but better, in line with your real needs and life goals. It's about getting out of the cycle of debt, impulse buying and instant gratification, and moving towards financial freedom, responsible choices and sustainable projects. This aspect of minimalism often leads to greater security, but above all to peace of mind.

Ultimately, modern minimalism is a philosophy of clarity and alignment. It does not dictate a single way of living, but offers a flexible framework for making better choices, living better and being better. It invites us to free ourselves of the unnecessary, to be silent around us and listen to what resonates within us. In this society that constantly pushes us to want more, minimalism whispers to us that the essential is already there if we take the time to see it.

The historical definition of Minimalism

The origins: an artistic movement that broke with the past

The term "minimalism" originated in contemporary art in the United States in the 1960s. It is not simply an aesthetic style, but first and foremost a critical response to the growing complexity of the art world at the time. Minimalism was a direct reaction against Abstract Expressionism, the predominant post-war movement, embodied by figures such as Jackson Pollock and Mark Rothko, in which the artist's subjectivity, raw emotion and gesture predominated. Faced with this emotional excess and the importance given to the artist's intention, the Minimalists proposed a new approach: stripping the work of all personal interpretation and reducing the artistic object to its most fundamental elements.

Artistic minimalism is based on formal reduction. It is characterised by the use of simple geometric forms, repetition, industrial materials (steel, Plexiglas, neon, concrete) and an often restricted palette of colours. The idea was to present the works in their raw material reality, with no hidden symbolism, no narrative, no overload. Artists such as Donald Judd, Carl Andre, Dan Flavin and Frank Stella played a major role in this aesthetic revolution. The viewer was no longer invited to interpret, but to experience the work in space, in its physicality. This marked a break with art as emotional discourse: the work became an autonomous object, often modular and repetitive, anchored in space.

Minimalism in architecture: the aesthetics of the essential

This artistic movement found a strong echo in the field of architecture architecture, where it was to take root and flourish. One of the pioneers of architectural minimalism was Ludwig Mies van der Rohe, a German-born architect who developed the idea that beauty comes from simplicity. His maxim "Less is more" became the mantra of architectural minimalism. This philosophy is based on pure volumes, noble and sober materials (glass, steel, raw concrete, light wood), straight lines and a strong desire for harmony between the building and its environment.

In this vision, each architectural element must have a raison d'être. The aim is not to create emptiness for emptiness's sake, but to design functional, airy, light-filled spaces where the superfluous is banished. The space becomes a source of serenity, a place that breathes. The absence of decoration is not a denial of aesthetics, but a conscious choice to essentialise: every detail counts, every material is highlighted by its simplicity. This minimalism has influenced generations of architects, notably in Japan with figures like Tadao Ando, who combines raw concrete, natural light and spirituality in his work.

From art to philosophy of life

From the 1980s to the 1990s, we witnessed a slow but profound transition: minimalism left the purely aesthetic field to infiltrate popular culture, design and then everyday life. This shift accelerated at the beginning of the 21st century. Against a backdrop of rampant globalisation, unbridled consumer growth, information overload and psychological exhaustion, more and more people are feeling oppressed by abundance. Possessing more does not necessarily bring more happiness. This disenchantment with consumer society is prompting some people to return t o forms of voluntary simplicity. This is where minimalism becomes a way of life in its own right.

Minimalism in life is inspired by this refined aesthetic, but gives it a practical and existential dimension. It's no longer just about creating simple objects or spaces, but about living simply. This means freeing ourselves from material, emotional and digital clutter. It means refusing to give in to the constant pressure to buy, to own, to appear. Many public figures, such as authors Joshua Fields Millburn and Ryan Nicodemus (known as The Minimalists), or Fumio Sasaki in Japan, have popularised this lifestyle by sharing their experiences: radical decluttering, reducing possessions to the essentials, returning to the essence of things.

A contemporary response to the excesses of modernity

Today, minimalism is a form of gentle resistance to the excesses of the modern world. It proposes a different way of living: slower, more conscious, more focused on the essentials. It questions our consumer habits and our relationship with objects, space and time. It invites us to return to ourselves, to a form of chosen sobriety, lucid and in line with our true needs and values.

In short, minimalism is a movement that has evolved from a radical artistic language into a global philosophy of life. It's no longer just about creating or owning less, but about living better, with less. This historical path shows that minimalism is not a passing fad, but a profound quest for meaning, born of a universal need to reconnect with the essential in a world saturated with demands.

Minimalism beyond decoration

To reduce minimalism to an aesthetic trend would be to miss its true nature. Of course, the sleek interiors in neutral colours, the functional furniture and tidy spaces that circulate on social networks can give a seductive first impression of this lifestyle. But minimalism is more than just stylish decoration or a passing fad. It's a profound philosophy of life, a daily intention, an art of simplifying for a better life. What we see on the surface - a pared-down interior, an organised cupboard, a capsule wardrobe - is only the outward manifestation of a much richer and more transformative inner process.

A lifestyle choice based on intention

At the heart of minimalism is a fundamental principle: living with intention. This means taking a clear-eyed look at what we own, what we do and what we think, and consciously choosing what to keep and what to discard. Minimalism encourages us to ask disturbing questions: Why did I buy this object? Does this activity really nourish me? Why am I in this relationship? What do I really want for my life? In this sense, it becomes a powerful tool for introspection and alignment with your deepest values.

Far from being a simple exercise in material sorting, minimalism is an inner process that frees us from social conditioning, automatisms, external expectations and even our own illusions. It invites us to take back control of our lives by letting go of all the clutter: useless objects, parasitic thoughts, non-essential obligations, harmful habits and toxic relationships. This opens up a new mental and emotional space, one that is conducive to clarity, creativity and personal fulfilment.

A response to modern overload

In our modern societies, saturated with consumer goods, information, digital stimuli, activities to do and goals to achieve, minimalism acts as a salutary counterweight. It encourages us to slow down, take a breath and regain control of our frenetic pace of life. All too often, we fill our days with fake emergencies, our homes with objects we never use, our thoughts with useless preoccupations. Minimalism suggests that we take a step aside and ask ourselves: what if I did less, but better?

This does not mean fleeing modernity or living like a hermit. Rather, it means rediscovering a form of personal sovereignty, learning to distinguish the necessary from the superfluous, the essential from the accessory. It means accepting not to do everything, not to have everything, not to follow everything, and in so doing rediscovering a precious freedom in a world that glorifies saturation and performance.

Minimalism in all areas of life

Applied in practical terms, minimalism can bring about profound changes in all areas of life:

- In time management: It encourages us to say no more often. No to pointless meetings, meaningless commitments and exhausting hobbies. It values the simplicity of routine, slowness and presence. It encourages you to create empty spaces where you can refocus, rest, dream or create. It reminds us that time is the only non-renewable resource, and that it deserves to be used wisely.

- Consumption: Minimalists don't seek deprivation, but awareness. They consume less, but better. They choose objects that are durable, repairable and useful. They reject impulse buying and trends dictated by advertising, and favour quality over quantity. His aim is not to own as little as possible, but to keep only what has real utility or emotional value.
- In relationships: Relationship minimalism is often overlooked, but it is fundamental. It means surrounding yourself with people who respect you, support you and inspire you. Sometimes it also means moving away from certain circles, cutting certain family or friendship ties that have become oppressive or toxic. A deep, sincere relationship is better than ten superficial, exhausting interactions.
- In our use of digital technology: Digital minimalism encourages us to sort out our information flows, unclutter our phones, limit our screen time and get out of the spiral of constant distraction. It suggests that we regain control of our attention, which is currently exploited by algorithms that fuel mental dispersion. By reverting to a sober, chosen approach to digital consumption, we can rediscover silence, concentration and serenity.
- At work: Minimalism can lead to career choices that are more in line with your deepest aspirations. This may involve refusing the race for promotion, changing career direction, or refocusing on a more modest but meaningful project. It's not the amount of responsibility or the prestige of the job that counts, but the consistency between what you do on a day-to-day basis and what you really are.

An invitation to inner freedom

Ultimately, minimalism is a philosophy of freedom. It frees up space, but above all it frees up the mind. It's not about living in a vacuum, but about creating space

space for what uplifts, soothes and inspires us. Everything in its place, every moment lived with attention, every relationship chosen with care: minimalism gives weight to every detail, flavour to every experience.

This lifestyle also teaches us the art of happy renunciation. Not as a sacrifice, but as a voluntary sorting out, a lucid refusal to accumulate in order to fill an inner void. The minimalist understands that this emptiness is precious, that it is the space in which joy, clarity, intuition and even true love are born.

By choosing a simpler life, we choose a fuller life. And therein lies the magnificent paradox of minimalism: it's not a loss, it's a gain. Not a gain in things, but a gain in life.

Myths and preconceived ideas

The myths of minimalism

An illusion shaped by contemporary society

In the age of social networking and aesthetic marketing, minimalism is often presented in a seductive, sleek, photogenic form. Instagram accounts, YouTube videos and documentaries featuring white, uncluttered, almost empty interiors have created a reductive and misleading image of minimalism. This dominant representation suggests that to live a minimalist lifestyle, you need to own very few things, live in a neutral, undecorated environment, with functional, impersonal furniture.

This visual myth becomes an implicit norm. It creates a silent pressure, especially among those who are discovering minimalism and looking for inspiration. In reality, this approach turns minimalism into a reverse consumer trend: instead of buying more, we try to throw everything away... sometimes without any real thought, just to achieve the perfect image. This is where the misunderstanding arises: minimalism is not an aesthetic to be imitated, but an approach to be lived.

Minimalism is not austerity

One of the most widespread misconceptions is that minimalism imposes a form of deprivation, an austerity akin to extreme stoicism. This view leads some people to believe that happiness can only be found in emptiness, that the slightest object kept would be a sign of failure, or even weakness. Yet this rigid interpretation totally misrepresents the essence of minimalism.

Being a minimalist does not mean living in lack, but rather living in the right. It means making room for what makes sense, for what sustains our well-being, for what nourishes our soul. It's not a question of giving up all material possessions, but of consciously choosing what we keep. A comfortable sofa, an inspiring painting, a collection of beloved books or a well-thought-out wardrobe can perfectly well be part of a minimalist life, as long as they are there for a clear reason, in line with our values.

True minimalist freedom does not come from the number of objects eliminated, but from the conscious relationship we have with what we own. It's not the number of objects that counts, but their relevance to our daily lives.

A personal path, not a universal rule

One of the most insidious traps in the myth of minimalism is the belief that there is only one way to be a minimalist, often inspired by iconic figures (bloggers, authors, influencers) who have turned this philosophy into a highly codified lifestyle. These figures sometimes give the impression that you have to follow their steps to the letter in order to live a 'good' minimalist life.

But this attitude is fundamentally contrary to the very spirit of Minimalism. This philosophy is based on freedom, personalisation and adaptation. Every human being has unique needs, desires, context and history. What is superfluous for one person may be essential for another. A musician may need several instruments, a photographer many accessories, a craftsman a workshop full of tools. All can be minimalists if they live with intention, without unnecessary excess or superfluous attachment.

Minimalism is not a fixed destination, but a process that is constantly evolving. It's an introspective process, a journey towards greater inner clarity and outer coherence. It's not about looking like someone else, but about living your own life to the full, on your own terms.

The perverse effects of the myth: stress, frustration, loss of bearings

Believing in the myth of minimalism can generate a form of symbolic violence against ourselves. By trying to simplify everything, we run the risk of falling into a minimalist perfectionism, a race for the purest detail that becomes an obsession. This desire to get rid of the superfluous can become a tyrannical objective, to the point of creating frustration, stress and even guilt when we keep an object that is important to us, or when we buy something out of need or pleasure.

There's also the risk of confusing the container with the content, of believing that the appearance of an uncluttered life guarantees a fulfilled life. But an empty house is not always synonymous with freedom; it can sometimes reflect an unacknowledged inner emptiness. Conversely, a lively, warm space can reflect a perfectly healthy minimalist balance. Minimalism does not judge appearance; it questions function and intention.

By focusing on rigid rules or numerical criteria (such as the number of objects), we forget the essential point: minimalism is there to serve us, not to constrain us. It's not a question of entering a new mental prison, but of getting out of the old ones.

Rediscovering the original meaning: simplifying for better living

Stripped of its modern distortions, minimalism rediscovers its nobility: that of a philosophy of life centred on the essentials. It encourages us to slow down, to sort things out, to refocus. It invites us to question our consumer automatisms, to move away from "always more" and towards "better". It gives us the opportunity to regain control of our attention, our energy and our time.

Minimalism doesn't ask us to own less for the sake of it, but t o own less in order to live better. Fewer useless objects often means more space, more mental clarity, more freedom of action. Fewer superfluous activities means more time for what really matters. Fewer distractions mean more presence. In this sense, minimalism becomes a tool for liberation, a path towards a fuller, more aligned, more conscious life.

Preconceived ideas about minimalism

The word 'minimalism' often conjures up stereotypical images: bare white interiors, people living with fewer than 100 objects, or almost ascetic individuals detached from the pleasures of life. This vision is reductive and creates a mental barrier for many people who could benefit from the principles of minimalism. It is therefore crucial to deconstruct these false beliefs in order to reveal the depth, flexibility and humanity of this approach.

Myth No. 1: "Minimalism means living with almost nothing".

This is probably the most widespread idea, and also the most distorting. Many people think that minimalism means reducing your life to the bare minimum, to the point of being almost uncomfortable. The minimalist is imagined as someone who sleeps on a futon, owns two T-shirts and a bowl, and rejects all material possessions as a source of harmful attachment. This vision, widely mediatised by viral challenges or extreme testimonials ("living with 50 objects", "a rucksack for life"), creates a rigid and inaccessible image of minimalism.

But this perception is profoundly mistaken. Minimalism is not defined by a quantity of objects, but by the subjective value we place on what we choose to keep. It's not about depriving yourself, but about freeing yourself from unnecessary clutter. Living with the essentials does not mean living in material poverty, but living with things that have meaning, real utility or genuine emotional value. The aim is not to have as little as possible, but to have just enough to live fully and serenely. And this measure is personal: what is superfluous for one person may be vital for another.

Myth No. 2: "Minimalism is an aesthetic trend".

Minimalism is often confused with aesthetics: immaculate interiors, white walls, light furniture, clean lines and a few carefully placed plants. This is the vision that dominates social networks and interior design magazines. Minimalism then becomes a visual code that we feel we have to adopt to be 'minimalist', which creates a form of silent pressure: if my home doesn't look like a Scandinavian version of an IKEA catalogue, then I'm 'out of the game'.

But minimalism is not a decorative style. Above all, it's a way of life. It's not about imitating a neutral, icy aesthetic, but about creating a space (and a life) that reflects your true needs, values and personality. An interior that is colourful, full of art or full of memories can be minimalist, if it is composed of elements chosen with care and meaning. The essence of minimalism lies not in beige tones or straight lines, but in the clarity of the choices you make, and in being consistent with yourself.

Myth no. 3: "Minimalism is for rich people".

Some critics claim that minimalism is a luxury reserved for those who can afford to "choose to have less", while others do not have this privilege. For them, minimalism is a posture of affluence, a choice reserved for those who have already had everything, and who can now afford to shed the superfluous while maintaining a financial and social safety net.

This ignores the reality of minimalism as a tool for emancipation. On the contrary, minimalism can help those who have little to live better with what they have, to disengage from the social pressure to consume, and to redirect their limited or scarce resources towards what really matters. It is a way out of the spiral of debt, over-consumption and waste. It teaches people to recognise the value of things before their price. And above all, it provides a structure

to regain control of your material life, even with limited means. This
It's not an elitist ideology, it's a universal tool for refocusing.

Myth No. 4: "Minimalists are cold, rigid and anti-social".

Minimalists are sometimes perceived as distant, almost misanthropic. We imagine them to be solitary, rigid, austere, cut off from human warmth, refusing any festivity or form of lightness in the name of an ideal of simplicity. This image may stem from a confusion between the search for order and emotional coldness, or from an overly monastic vision of renunciation.

But minimalism doesn't cut you off from the world, it reconnects you with it. By reducing distractions, unnecessary commitments and cumbersome possessions, it opens up time and space for what's essential, and this essential is often made up of relationships, emotions and human sharing. A minimalist may well be someone who is extremely warm, generous and deeply connected to others, precisely because they have chosen not to disperse their energy in the superficial. They don't reject connections; they choose them consciously and honour them authentically.

Myth no. 5: "Minimalism will automatically make me happy".

A subtle but dangerous belief has crept into some popular discourse: minimalism is the miracle solution to modern malaise. All you have to do is sort out your home, throw out some boxes, simplify your commitments and unclutter your cupboards to finally find inner peace, mental clarity and emotional serenity.

But that's forgetting that minimalism is a tool, not a magic solution. It can offer conditions conducive to well-being, but it doesn't solve everything. Decluttering your flat won't heal a deep emotional wound.

Emptying your dressing room doesn't erase feelings of loneliness. Reducing your possessions does not automatically cancel out anxiety or inner conflicts. On the other hand, minimalism creates a space conducive to introspection, self-discovery and reflection on our true priorities. It makes it easier to get to the root of our discomforts, but it doesn't do the work for us. It's a starting point, not an end point.

Why do these preconceived ideas persist?

The persistence of these preconceived ideas can be explained by the way minimalism is presented in the media. Radical approaches are more 'saleable', more 'Instagrammable'. An empty, white flat attracts more attention than a subtle, nuanced interior story. What's more, image culture favours visible results over inner evolution. It's not so easy to show a calmer, more present, more aligned person as it is to show a decluttered room.

Finally, our society is still deeply attached to materialism: owning things is still a marker of social success. Questioning this can be upsetting, provoke scepticism, or be derided. Hence the mistrust, snap judgements and caricatures. But when we go beyond these filters, we discover a minimalism that is much more human, benevolent and transformative than we imagine.

Preconceived ideas about minimalism create a smokescreen between us and a practice that could profoundly improve our daily lives. In truth, minimalism doesn't impose anything: it invites. It doesn't judge: it questions. It doesn't reduce life: it lightens it to better reveal its richness. By stripping it of its clichés, we can finally discover it for what it really is: an art of living founded on freedom, awareness and coherence.

Chapter 2: The benefits of minimalism

Mental and emotional clarity

Adopting a minimalist approach to life isn't just about decluttering your physical space; it's also an inner process, a transformation that directly affects the way you think, feel and live. Minimalism acts as a filter, a sieve through which we can sort not only objects, but also thoughts, emotions, relationships and commitments. By removing the superfluous and refocusing on the essential, we allow our minds to regain clarity and our emotions to breathe. This process leads to much greater inner stability than we might imagine.

1. The direct impact of our environment on our mental state

The environment in which we live acts as a mirror of our inner world. When it is overloaded, chaotic or full of useless objects, it provokes constant stimulation of the brain. Every object in sight, every pile of papers, every misplaced drawer is an unspoken demand for attention. Unconsciously, these items remind us of tasks to be carried out, decisions to be made and memories that are sometimes heavy. This overloads our minds with silent signals, creating a permanent mental fog.

In contrast, when the space is uncluttered, fluid and functional, the brain relaxes. There are fewer visual distractions, less information to process. Calm on the outside becomes an extension of calm on the inside. A minimalist space does not mean empty or cold, but it is deliberate: every object has a place and a purpose.

purpose. This intentionality is reflected in the way we think. External order facilitates internal order.

2. Reducing decision fatigue

Every day we make between 35,000 and 50,000 micro-decisions, w h e t h e r it's choosing what to eat, what to wear, what task to start or what message to respond to. This leads to what psychologists call "decision fatigue": the more decisions we make, the more exhausted our brains become, and the more difficult it becomes to make relevant choices. Minimalism drastically reduces this background noise. Having fewer but carefully chosen clothes means avoiding an internal debate every morning about the ideal outfit. Having fewer gadgets means less wondering which tool to use for which task.

By reducing the options available, minimalism saves mental energy for the really important decisions. It frees us from the tyranny of choice. This cognitive economy translates into a feeling of mental lightness, clarity and fluidity in everyday life. We become more efficient, more creative and less stressed when faced with the unexpected.

3. Freeing up emotional space: lightening the heart and mind

Beyond material possessions, minimalism suggests sorting out our emotional attachments. Many of our possessions are linked to memories, people or past moments. These objects can harbour painful attachments, heavy nostalgia and even a form of unconscious self-sabotage. By keeping certain objects 'just in case', or out of fear of missing out, we maintain a toxic emotional relationship with the past or fear of the future.

Minimalism invites us to free ourselves of this unnecessary emotional burden. It's not about denying our memories or emotions, but about choosing what we really want to carry with us. Each object that is eliminated becomes a form of healthy mourning, an affirmation that we are moving forward. And each freed-up space becomes an invitation to renewal. So minimalism doesn't empty us: it opens us up. It makes our inner world more spacious, more peaceful, more available to what really matters.

4. Reconstructing identity from the essentials

Modern consumerism pushes us to define our value through what we possess: our appearance, our status, our technology, our networks. Minimalism proposes a reversal: we are not what we own, but what we live, what we cultivate, what we embody. This redefinition of identity gives us immense emotional freedom. By ceasing to chase after objects or external signs of success, we find the time, space and energy to explore who we really are.

This quest for meaning, facilitated by our new-found mental clarity, encourages us to align our actions with our deepest values. We become less reactive to fads, external judgements and social comparisons. This inner stability, nurtured by a simplified lifestyle, enables us to develop genuine emotional intelligence. We better understand what we feel, why we feel it, and how to respond appropriately.

5. Cultivating presence, mindfulness and inner peace

Finally, the mental and emotional clarity that comes from minimalism is a gateway to mindfulness. By removing material and mental distractions, we become more present to what we are experiencing. You eat by tasting, you talk by listening, you walk by observing. The mind is no longer constantly occupied by futile preoccupations. This self-presence, supported by a calm environment, fosters lasting peace. With less pressure on the mind, the spirit can rest, and emotions can flow freely without being repressed or amplified.

Minimalism, far from being a mere aesthetic or fashion statement, becomes a genuine form of psychological and emotional hygiene. It teaches us to distinguish the essential from the accessory, to cultivate gratitude for what we have, and to create an inner space conducive to serenity and lucidity.

Reducing stress and anxiety

In a modern society marked by hyperstimulation, a constantly accelerating pace of life and a culture of mass consumption, stress and anxiety have become commonplace, almost commonplace ailments. Minimalism is a radically different response: it does not seek to mask these tensions with distractions or compensations, but to eradicate their root cause by simplifying our environment, our thoughts and our behaviour. Contrary to the generally accepted idea that minimalism is a form of deprivation, it is in fact an art of living that aims to free the individual from everything that clutters him or her up unnecessarily materially, emotionally and mentally, in order to regain a deep sense of calm, clarity and control.

1. The calming effect of empty space

Visual overload in living spaces - piles of papers, piles of clothes, forgotten objects on furniture, knick-knacks t h a t accumulate without coherence - has a calming effect on the mind.

direct impact on the brain. It is constantly called upon to interpret, analyse and evaluate what it sees. Even if we are not always aware of it, a cluttered environment creates 'visual noise' that interferes with our ability to concentrate and relax. Simply walking through a disorganised room can activate vigilance circuits in our autonomic nervous system, raising our levels of the stress hormone cortisol. Conversely, a minimalist, uncluttered, breathable interior sends a signal of safety and peace to the brain. There's nothing to monitor, nothing to manage, nothing to sort through mentally. The empty space becomes a mental space. It creates a sensation of lightness, almost physical, that instantly relaxes internal tensions.

2. Decluttering to free the mind

Every object has an implicit memory and a psychic charge. A book never read recalls an unfinished task. A piece of clothing never worn echoes an idealised version of ourselves. An unwanted gift refers to a social or emotional obligation. So behind every possession lies a micro-narrative that engages our minds. This phenomenon is subtle, but cumulative. As objects pile up, our mental load increases, often without us being able to identify the cause. By decluttering, the minimalist doesn't just part with physical objects: he or she also breaks with psychological attachments, regrets from the past, unrealistic expectations or emotional obligations. They consciously choose to let go in order to feel lighter, freer and more centred. This process, although uncomfortable at first, triggers a profound sense of relief. The less you own, the more your mind is freed from latent tensions.

3. Simplify to reduce decision fatigue

Every day, we are faced with a multitude of decisions: what to wear? What to eat? What to watch? What to do tonight? When there are too many of these choices create what is known as decision fatigue. Even seemingly innocuous decisions, such as choosing between ten shirts or twenty types of cereal, can exhaust our mental resources. This fatigue reduces our capacity for concentration, patience and tolerance - all factors that aggravate anxiety. Minimalism, by deliberately limiting the number of options available, relieves this pressure considerably. A dressing room reduced to the essentials, for example, avoids wasting time each morning putting together an outfit. A minimalist kitchen avoids waste, hesitation and compulsions. This simplification has a direct effect on stress levels: less choice = less stress = more energy for what really matters.

4. A calmer pace of life, far from the constant rush

Minimalism isn't just about material possessions, it's also a philosophy of slowing down. By refusing to submit to the overloaded agenda dictated by a society of ever more work, leisure, travel and notifications, the minimalist chooses to take back control of his or her time. They stop filling up every minute of the day as if they had to make the most of it. They learn to say no to superfluous demands, empty commitments and toxic or energy-guzzling relationships. This refusal of overactivity is not a retreat, but a reconquest. It allows us to make time for calm, rest and solitude in our daily lives. These moments of silence are essential for lowering physiological stress levels, regulating the nervous system and encouraging a return to oneself. Modern stress also comes from our inability to stop. Minimalists stop. They breathe. They observe. They feel.

5. A life refocused on the emotional essentials

When you declutter your space and your schedule, you create a fertile void: a space in which real needs, real desires and deep emotions can emerge. Minimalism acts like a filter: it eliminates the superfluous to reveal the essential.

the superfluous to reveal the essential. And this essential, very often, has nothing to do with possessions or performance. It's found in simple but fundamental things: a sincere relationship, a walk in nature, a home-cooked meal, a moment of silence, a good book, a look, a smile. By reconnecting with these elements, we reconnect with ourselves. We relieve the internal tensions created by social comparison, the pressure to succeed, the quest for image. Stress often stems from a gap between what we are experiencing and what we think we should be experiencing. Minimalism fills this gap by bringing us back to what is right, sufficient and nourishing.

6. Fewer obligations, more control

The accumulation of objects and commitments creates a multiplication of obligations. You have to maintain, tidy up, repair, pay off, organise and manage. It all adds up to a life full of constant micro-stress. Minimalism, by reducing the number of material and social commitments, allows us to regain a sense of control over our own lives. This feeling of being in control is fundamental to calming anxiety. You no longer feel like a victim of circumstances or a prisoner of your possessions. You become an active, conscious and intentional player again. Every object is chosen. Every relationship is carefully nurtured. Every action has meaning. This refocusing gives you inner stability, a solid foundation that helps you to face life's inevitable challenges without becoming overwhelmed.

7. An antidote to performance anxiety

Finally, minimalism is also a response to the omnipresent anxiety about having to
Finally, minimalism is also a response to the omnipresent fear of having to "succeed in life" according to criteria imposed from outside: wealth, appearance, status, number of subscribers. This constant pressure to do more, be more, show more, is one of the main generators of modern anxiety. Minimalism challenges these injunctions. It asserts that the value of a life is not measured by accumulation but by coherence. A simple, sober life

values, can be infinitely more satisfying and calming than a life that is brilliant on the surface but chaotic on the inside. By detaching themselves from this logic of performance, the minimalist regains the right to be imperfect, slow and human. And this assumed humanity, far removed from social masks, is a profound source of peace.

Saving time, money and energy

When fully understood and integrated, minimalism becomes much more than a simple aesthetic choice or a trendy lifestyle. It's a profoundly transformative philosophy that aims to free people from the burden of excess, enabling them to regain what modern society all too often causes them to lose: control over their time, money and energy. In a world saturated with stimuli, advertising, useless objects and artificial social obligations, minimalism proposes a return to the essentials. This deliberately simplifying approach creates tangible gains in these three fundamental dimensions of human life.

1. Saving time: the most underestimated resource

Time is the one resource that we cannot buy back, extend or make up for once it has been lost. Yet it is the one resource we most often waste. Minimalism allows us to reclaim this precious time by freeing us from micro-tasks, distractions, unaligned social commitments and time-consuming possessions.

Let's take a simple example: owning a wardrobe of 100 pieces versus a capsule wardrobe of 20 carefully chosen pieces. Every morning, the decision of

"What to wear" becomes a source of avoided stress. This concept, known as decision fatigue, shows that the more options we have, the more we use our mental energy and time on trivial choices. Minimalism reduces this decision-making noise and frees up mental time for what's really important.

Beyond the personal sphere, this time-saving extends to all spheres of life: less time cleaning objects, looking for things, organising useless things, returning impulse purchases, solving problems related to non-essential possessions. Even our leisure time becomes more intentional: instead of spending hours shopping or scrolling through consumer apps, the time saved can be used for fulfilling activities, such as reading, creating, reconnecting with nature, or simply doing nothing - the ultimate luxury in a society of constant hustle and bustle.

2. Saving money: Spend less to live better

One of the most visible effects of minimalism is reduced spending. By adopting a posture of voluntary sobriety, we learn to differentiate between real need and temporary desire. Modern marketing is cleverly designed to create an illusion of lack: we think we need the latest gadget, the latest trend or that thing that everyone else has. Minimalism shatters this illusion and teaches us to ask a fundamental question before every purchase: "Does this really add value to my life?"

By drastically reducing unnecessary purchases, we start to realise just how much we've been manipulated. It's not just a one-off saving, but a complete transformation of our relationship with money. Less shopping also means less debt, fewer instalments, less consumer credit, and therefore greater financial peace of mind. You realise that an object you don't buy doesn't need to be stored, cleaned, insured, repaired or replaced, repaired or replaced. Each expense avoided frees up an invisible chain of responsibilities.

This financial freedom can then be used more strategically: saving for meaningful projects, investing in personal development, building up a security reserve, or even reducing your working hours. Minimalism is not a miserly or restrictive approach, but a strategy for consciously allocating resources. It's about doing more with less, and returning money to its role as a tool for life, rather than an all-powerful master.

3. Save energy: less mental workload, more vitality

One of the most insidious consequences of an overloaded lifestyle is the dissipation of mental, physical and emotional energy. By chasing after possessions, status and appearances, our minds are constantly stretched, fragmented and parasitised. Minimalism acts here as a genuine refocusing therapy.

Fewer objects in the environment means less visual clutter, and therefore less unnecessary cognitive stimulation. This phenomenon, studied in neuroscience, shows that clutter is directly linked to an increase in cortisol, the stress hormone. Conversely, an uncluttered, calm, breathable space encourages relaxation, concentration and mental clarity. It's no coincidence that monasteries and meditation centres are essentially minimalist.

On a physical level, minimalism also lightens the load. There's less to carry, less to move and less to manage on a daily basis. The result is a general feeling of lightness, as if invisible weights had been lifted. You can even see it in your diary: fewer superficial social obligations, fewer appointments dictated by the desire to please or the fear of missing out. The energy you gain allows you to redirect your attention to what really nourishes your soul: your family, your health, your spirituality, your creativity.

Finally, on an emotional level, living a minimalist lifestyle reduces social comparison, envy and feelings of failure. By detaching ourselves from external standards, we stop measuring our value in terms of what we have. You reconnect with yourself. This saving o f inner energy is priceless: it's a return t o serenity.

Minimalism isn't just about making space in your cupboards. It's profoundly liberating: it gives us back time to live, money to choose, and energy to create, love, rest and think. These resources, once recovered, enable us to build a more aligned, clearer and happier life. It's not a loss, it's a gain. It's not a restriction, it's an expansion. Minimalism is not a sacrifice: it is an intentional rebirth.

Ecological and social impact

In a world where hyper-consumption has become a cultural and economic norm, minimalism represents much more than an aesthetic or personal choice: it is a lucid and committed response to the ecological and social crises that are shaking our times. By advocating voluntary simplicity and happy sobriety, the minimalist lifestyle has a transformative impact on our relationship with objects, the environment, others and even ourselves. It acts as a powerful lever for systemic change, at the ecological, economic and societal levels.

1. A lifestyle that reduces our ecological footprint

One of the most direct consequences of minimalism is the massive reduction in the individual's environmental footprint. Against a backdrop of climate change, dwindling natural resources and the collapse of biodiversity, adopting a lifestyle based on the essentials becomes a profoundly ecological act. By reducing their purchases and favouring sustainability over quantity, minimalists limit the overall demand for consumer goods. This translates into less industrial production, so less resource extraction, fewer CO_2 emissions, less pollution, less transport, and less waste.

For example, choosing to buy one quality, ethical and sustainable garment rather than ten cheap items produced in dubious fast fashion conditions not only reduces the number o f purchases, but also implicitly rejects a system based on the exploitation of the environment and human beings. Minimalism encourages us to think about the origin, lifespan and end of each item we buy, which in turn encourages responsible practices such as buying locally, buying second-hand, repairing and recycling. Every purchase becomes a conscious act aligned with strong ecological values.

2. A break with the destructive logic of over-consumption

Contemporary society is based on unlimited economic growth, fuelled by the constant and often compulsive consumption of goods and services. While this model has brought unprecedented material comfort, it is now recognised as being unsustainable, both ecologically and in human terms. Ubiquitous advertising, programmed obsolescence, the pressure of fashion and social networks all contribute to a culture of excessive consumption, where "having more" is confused with "being more".

Minimalism proposes a silent but radical revolution: that of voluntary degrowth. It invites us to break out of the cycle of desire, purchase, possession, frustration and replacement that fuels contemporary capitalism. By ceasing to consume to fill emotional gaps or to conform to social expectations, the minimalist breaks with a spiral of dependency and waste. This lifestyle choice is not a withdrawal into oneself, but an act of joyful resistance in the face of an economic model that is destroying the planet while generating a growing sense of unease among individuals.

3. Encouraging relocation and a humane economy

Minimalism not only rejects over-consumption, it also encourages a more humane and local economy. By valuing quality over quantity, short supply chains over mass imports, craftsmanship over impersonal industrial production, it supports economic players who respect ecological and social values. Buying something made locally, ethically, not only limits transport-related emissions, but also promotes local employment, transparency and decent working conditions.

This change in consumer behaviour is far from insignificant: it is part of a reconfiguration of economic flows. It empowers citizen-consumers to encourage responsible, ethical and sustainable businesses. Minimalism thus becomes a tool for ecological and social transition, supporting an economy rooted in solidarity, proximity and respect for living things. It embodies a vision of wealth that is measured not by the accumulation of goods, but by the quality of human exchanges, balance with nature and inner peace.

4. Challenging inequalities and social norms

In a society where material possession is often synonymous with success, minimalism offers a powerful deconstruction of dominant social norms. It encourages us to detach our identity and personal value from the objects we own. This has profound social repercussions: the minimalist refuses to play the game of social competition through consumption. They free themselves from the need to "appear", to "possess in order to exist", and value being over having.

This ethical stance calls into question the social inequalities exacerbated by consumerism. Where some people sink into debt to maintain an image or an artificial lifestyle, the minimalist chooses conscious, liberating and accessible frugality. This does not mean living in want, but living in accordance with your real needs, far from excess and superfluous. Minimalism then becomes a factor of social justice: it puts everyone on an equal footing, because it values intention, balance and awareness rather than purchasing power or social status.

5. Fertile ground for solidarity and collective transformation

Finally, minimalism goes beyond the individual sphere to affect the collective. It is often accompanied by a desire for sharing, mutualisation and sobriety. By freeing ourselves from superfluous material possessions, we discover that we have more to offer: time, energy, listening and attention. Minimalists tend to open up to others, joining circles where resources, skills and ideas are shared. This can take the form of recycling centres, object libraries, donation groups, repair workshops, volunteering or community life.

In this context, minimalism becomes a powerful engine for social transformation. It fosters the resilience of local communities, strengthens the social fabric and gives new meaning to mutual aid. It also helps to build a fairer, more sustainable future, where everyone's needs are met without compromising those of others or of future generations.

Far from being a simple lifestyle trend, minimalism is a philosophy of life with far-reaching personal and collective implications. Its ecological impact can be seen in the reduction of our carbon footprint, the preservation of resources and the fight against pollution. Its social impact lies in transforming our relationship to consumption, challenging unequal social norms and rebuilding more authentic human ties. Adopting minimalism means making the courageous choice to live differently, in harmony with the planet and with others, in a spirit of responsibility, lucidity and freedom.

Chapter 3: The roots of clutter

Consumerism and the society of overabundance

A system based on accumulation: the heart of the problem

Modern consumerism is an economic and cultural model based on the idea that happiness, success and personal fulfilment depend on the constant acquisition of material goods. This paradigm has taken deep root in industrialised societies, particularly since the 20th century with the rise of mass production. The more we consume, the more the economy grows, and the more this cycle is encouraged by companies, institutions and the media. It's no longer just a question of satisfying vital or utilitarian needs, but of constantly creating new desires.

new desires. Advertising plays a fundamental role here: it persuades us that what we have is never enough, that something is always missing, and that this object in the shop window or on our screen is perhaps the solution to that lack.

So consumerism is more than just buying behaviour. It is a subtle and powerful mental conditioning. It shapes our choices, our relationship with ourselves and with others. It encourages us to define our personal value in terms of what we own: the brand of our phone, the style of our home, the size of our wardrobe. This logic creates a never-ending dynamic where "more and more" becomes the norm. Even after buying a product, a new version, an improvement or an emerging trend quickly relegates the old one to technical or social obsolescence. This cycle fuels chronic dissatisfaction and a headlong rush into the future.

Material glut: illusion of freedom, source of disorder

In a society where goods are accessible in abundance, often at low cost, the act of buying has become trivial. We can order at any time, from anywhere, with just a few clicks. Instantaneity and ease of access reinforce impulsive behaviour. We buy more than we need, often without thinking. Promotions, sales and flash sales create an artificial sense of urgency that drives us to accumulate more. As a result, our living spaces fill up at a much faster rate than our real needs.

This overabundance has an invisible but very real price. The material clutter that insidiously creeps into our homes creates physical, as well as emotional and mental, clutter. Every object takes up space, needs attention, and needs to be looked after, tidied up and moved. Even unused or forgotten objects affect us unconsciously: they clutter up our visual field,

our environment and create a constant background noise in our minds.
noise in our minds. Our living space becomes crowded, oppressive and fragmented. It no longer breathes.

And yet, in a world where everything moves so fast, space should be a place to recharge our batteries. All too often, it becomes a place of accumulation, saturation and even guilt. We keep things 'just in case', gifts we don't like but don't dare throw away, clothes we no longer wear but hope to wear again one day. We live surrounded by 'too much': too many options, too many duplicates, too many traces of the past. This affects our well-being, our mental clarity and our ability to concentrate on what really matters.

The illusion of happiness through possession

One of the foundations of consumerism is the association between possession and happiness. This deeply rooted idea is omnipresent in media stories, social networks, films and advertising. We are shown that a successful life means owning a beautiful house, an elegant car and a luxurious wardrobe. But behind this promise of happiness lies a very different reality: once the object has been acquired, the pleasure felt is often fleeting. We experience what psychologists call "hedonic adaptation": what excited us yesterday quickly becomes commonplace. Euphoria gives way to habit, then to a new need to be filled.

This mechanism creates an endless loop of consumption: we buy to feel, then we consume again to regain that lost sensation. Happiness becomes conditional on purchase, and the absence of something new is perceived as a void. This constant quest for things to make us feel better often masks a deeper need: for recognition, love, security a n d meaning. But as long as these needs are not consciously identified and nurtured, consumption continues to act as a temporary emotional band-aid.

Clutter then becomes the visible symptom of a deeper malaise. Behind every drawer full of useless objects, every overflowing cupboard, there is often an unconscious attempt to fill an inner void. Understanding this dynamic is already a step towards a more aligned, clearer life.

Minimalism: a conscious response to overabundance

Minimalism is not opposed to consumption as such, but to unconscious, excessive consumption dictated by the outside world. It proposes to reverse the logic of consumerism by rehabilitating the value of the essential. Where the world says "more", minimalism says "better". It invites us to question each possession: does it bring me value? Does it correspond to my deepest needs, priorities and aspirations? This process of conscious selection transforms our relationship with objects, but also with ourselves. We stop identifying with what we own and start rooting ourselves in what we experience, what we feel, what we are.

Choosing minimalism does not mean giving up all forms of comfort or material beauty. It means choosing quality over quantity, sustainability over the ephemeral, alignment over conformity. It means rediscovering a feeling of clarity, lightness and freedom. Because by freeing ourselves f r o m physical clutter, we also free up mental space, energy and time. You regain control over your environment, but also over your life.

So, by understanding that our clutter is not simply due to a lack of organisation, but to a wider social and psychological logic, we can take a critical look at the prevailing consumerism. This is the first step towards a lasting transformation: one that leads to a simpler life, but one that is infinitely richer in meaning.

Emotional attachments to objects

A deep and silent root of clutter

Clutter is not just an accumulation of useless or untidy objects. It is often the material reflection of much more subtle inner processes, rooted in our history, our psychology and our emotional wounds. Among these roots, emotional attachment to objects is undoubtedly one of the most powerful and unconscious factors preventing us from decluttering our living space.

When objects become emotional receptacles

Every object we keep has an emotional history, sometimes light-hearted, sometimes deeply rooted. A simple T-shirt can evoke an unforgettable summer. An old, worn handbag may be linked to our first professional success. A battered book may represent a time in our lives when we felt alive, in love, free or creative.

This phenomenon is perfectly human: our brains are wired to create associations between things and experiences. Objects then become symbolic receptacles for memories, bridges to the past, anchors of identity that remind us of who we were, where we've been, and sometimes even who we'd like to have become.

But the problem starts when these emotional associations take over our ability to make rational choices. We no longer see the object as a lifeless piece of matter, but as we feel it inside. The object becomes sacred, almost inviolable, even if it is damaged, useless or cumbersome.

The invisible weight of guilt and emotional duty

Very often, emotional attachment is reinforced, even contaminated, by a feeling of guilt. It's not just a question of remembrance, but also of implicit loyalty to the people who gave us these objects or to past versions of ourselves. We say to ourselves:

- "I can't throw this jumper away, my grandmother knitted it for me."
- "It was my ex who gave it to me, even though it hurts, it reminds me that he mattered."
- "I spent a lot of money on it, even if I never use it, I can't throw it away. throw it away."
- "It's a memory of my childhood, it's part of me."

Guilt creeps in everywhere. It creates an emotional obligation to keep something that has nothing to do with the actual usefulness of the object. We no longer keep objects because they do us a favour, but because we believe that by parting with them we are betraying something or someone. This invisible link chains us to a frozen and sometimes painful past. As a result, our home becomes an emotional mausoleum rather than a living space adapted to our present needs.

Identity projected through objects

Another aspect of emotional attachment is the illusion of identity that objects construct or preserve. We keep books that we will never read, but which give us the image of a cultured person. We keep clothes from another era, another style, another size, in the hope (or illusion) of becoming that idealised version of ourselves again. We stockpile sports equipment or musical instruments to maintain the idea that we are 'active', 'curious' or 'curious'.

are 'active', 'curious', 'versatile', even if these objects are never used.

These possessions become the remnants of past or fantasised identities. They don't serve our current needs, but feed an inner narrative, often unconscious, about who we think we are or who we'd like to become. And as long as we don't question these narratives, we remain prisoners of these objects that freeze our evolution.

The "just in case" syndrome

One of the most insidious faces of emotional attachment is the fear of missing out or regretting something. This reflex, commonly known as "just in case", is one of the major obstacles to decluttering. It's based on an implicit belief that the item could be used one day, even if that day has never come in years.

This fear often stems from a scarcity mentality: fear of not being able to buy, of not having the means, of lacking resources or solutions. It can also reflect a fear of insecurity, inherited from a strict upbringing, a childhood marked by scarcity or a financial trauma. So we keep five can-openers, useless cables, out-of-season clothes, broken objects and duplicates, simply "just in case".

The paradox is that this need for security leads us to accumulate useless items that weigh down our daily lives. It generates physical and mental clutter: each surplus object becomes an unconscious micro-stress, a silent reminder of decisions not taken.

freeing up without betraying your memory

A common mistake is to believe that parting with an object is tantamount to forgetting what it represents. But memory is not contained in objects: it is contained within us. Our memories, our learning and our emotions are part of our personal history. Throwing away a dress doesn't make the love you felt when wearing it disappear. Giving away a trinket doesn't erase the link with a departed person.

Symbolic rituals can be used to gently let go. By
for example:

- Photograph the objects before giving them away.
- Write a letter to a person whose physical memory you are parting with.
- Create an intentional memory box, limited in size, to keep only the essentials.
- Give the objects to someone who will need them, to transform them into a lasting memory.

  attachment into a gesture of transmission.

These gestures help to transform the mourning of the object into a conscious, calmed act, respectful of oneself and one's history.

Decluttering as an act of self-love

Finally, understanding emotional attachments to objects helps t o reconcile minimalism with kindness. It's not about forcing yourself to live with three T-shirts and two spoons. It's about learning to distinguish between what we keep out of love and usefulness, and what we keep out of fear, guilt or illusion.

Decluttering is not about throwing things away for the sake of throwing them away. It's about honouring what's important, and then
making the choice to live in the present, with what nourishes us today. It's about

an act of lucidity and maturity, but also of profound love for ourselves: by freeing ourselves from the emotional weight of objects, we make room for clarity, creativity, inner peace and personal evolution.

Our environment then becomes a faithful reflection of who we are now, rather than a frozen museum of what we once were.

Fear of lack and boredom

Clutter in our lives doesn't just manifest itself in the visible accumulation of objects. Above all, it stems from fertile psychological ground, fed by deep-seated, unconscious fears. Among these fears, two are particularly active and formidable: the fear of lack and the fear of boredom. These are powerful drivers of our hoarding habits. As long as they are not identified, understood and allayed, these fears will continue to encourage excessive consumption and an inability to let go of the superfluous, making any attempt at minimalism unstable or superficial.

1. Fear of lack: the "just in case" fantasy

Fear of lack is often rooted in a life experience marked by insecurity, whether real or perceived. It is intimately linked to our survival instinct. Humans have always had to plan for periods of scarcity, cold or danger. This reflex of storage and foresight was vital in contexts where resources were scarce or unpredictable. But in a modern world where material abundance is instantly accessible, this mechanism, which remains active in our subconscious, often becomes dysfunctional.

Many people have kept objects, clothes, utensils, papers or gadgets in their homes for years simply "just in case". This simple expression, seemingly banal, actually conceals an anxiety: the fear of not having what they need when an unforeseen situation arises. Behind this fear lies a deep-seated need for security, control over the future and emotional reassurance. The worst thing is that the more we accumulate "to feel ready", the more we feel overwhelmed, encumbered, suffocated and, paradoxically, even more insecure.

This reflex is reinforced by our cultural and economic environment. Marketing plays on this fear by convincing us that the object we don't yet own could one day be sorely missed. Limited offers, sales, emergency messages such as "last in stock" or "don't miss this opportunity" are designed to awaken this fear of missing out, of not being equipped, of not being ready. So we accumulate far more out of precaution than utility. We keep clothes that are too small, broken appliances, out-of-date textbooks... not because we need them, but because one day, perhaps, they could be used again.

But this fear of lack is deceptive. It makes us believe that the object is our lifeline, when in reality it's our ability to adapt, our creativity, our social network, or our capacity to ask for help that will save us in a difficult situation. Minimalism proposes an inner revolution: it invites us to rebuild a deep trust in ourselves and in life, to believe that we will have what we need, when we need it, not because we have stored everything up, but because we have developed the inner resources to cope.

2. Fear of boredom: the compulsive need to fill up

If the fear of lack is focused on the future - "I might need it one day" - the fear of boredom is focused on the future - "I might need it one day".
the fear of boredom is a reaction to the present. In a saturated world

boredom has become almost unbearable. And yet boredom is a natural and healthy state, an empty space necessary for creativity, introspection and mental rest. But many people dread it. For some, boredom is associated with loneliness, uselessness, or even an agonising existential void. So they run away from it, not by going back to what's essential, but by surrounding themselves with material distractions.

This fear of boredom leads us to multiply our possessions in the illusion of filling an inner void. We buy things we don't really need, we stockpile potential activities such as unread books, instruments we've never played and unused leisure equipment, as if the accumulation of options would save us from a momentary slump. The house then becomes a museum of unfinished projects. Each object is an unfulfilled promise, a silent reminder that we are trying to escape ourselves through the outside world.

Fear of boredom also leads us to confuse being busy with being alive. We believe that by filling every space, every moment, we avoid the anguish of feeling nothing, doing nothing, being *nobody*. In reality, this overflow prevents us from finding ourselves. It creates noise, confusion and agitation. It becomes difficult to concentrate, to feel gratitude, or simply to be at peace with the present moment.

Minimalism teaches us an essential lesson here: emptiness is precious. It's in empty spaces that we breathe, that light enters, that thought is ordered. It is in the silences that profound ideas are born. By learning t o accept boredom, to tame it, we stop trying to escape it through consumption. We discover that behind boredom lies an opportunity: the chance to reconnect with ourselves, to explore our true emotions, thoughts and desires.

3. Hoarding as an emotional avoidance strategy

These two fears of lack and boredom have the same function in common
to avoid confronting an inner vulnerability. Clutter then becomes armour. It gives the illusion of a world under control, of a well-filled life, whereas it often masks a deeper malaise. Hoarding is sometimes an attempt to fill an emotional void, compensate for a lack of love, escape existential angst or avoid inner discomfort.

Objects then become extensions of our unprocessed emotions. That old piece of clothing kept in a drawer evokes a memory we don't want to give up. That drawer full of gadgets distracts us from our professional dissatisfaction. That pile of unread books gives us the illusion that we're still on our way to something. As long as we don't look these fears in the face, we'll continue to feed them, not by appeasing them, but by dressing them up.

4. Minimalism as psychological healing

Adopting minimalism is first and foremost a matter of inner work. It's not just about throwing things away or tidying up more efficiently, but about deconstructing the beliefs and fears that have driven us to accumulate. It's an act of reconciliation with emptiness, with the present moment, with ourselves. It requires courage: the courage to confront our insecurities, to observe our automatisms, to resist the call of illusory comfort.

By facing up to the fear of lack, we discover that true security lies not in possessions, but in clarity, simplicity and autonomy. By taming the fear of boredom, we discover that emptiness is not an enemy, but a sacred space where we can finally *be*, without the need to justify ourselves, to occupy ourselves or to consume.

Fear of lack and fear of boredom are deep-seated conditioning. They trap us in a vicious circle of accumulation and overload. Minimalism, properly understood, is not about emptying things out to look pretty: it's a b o u t freeing up space to live better. It invites us to move from a logic of possession to a logic of presence. To choose what's essential. To make peace with uncertainty and silence. Because it's precisely in these empty spaces that we find freedom, clarity and the joy of living with less but better.

Part II - Applying Minimalism to Everyday Life

Chapter 4: Simplifying your space

De-clutter effectively (KonMari, 90/90 methods, etc.)

De-cluttering is not simply a matter of tidying up or aesthetics: it's an inner, almost spiritual process, which consists of regaining power over our physical environment in order to better control our inner world. In an age dominated by over-consumption, persuasive marketing and excessive possessions, our space becomes a reflection of our mental state. An overloaded environment generates stress, constant mental fatigue and even a form of diffuse anxiety. Conversely, an uncluttered living space, organised and thought through with intention, becomes a sanctuary of peace and concentration.

De-cluttering effectively means freeing ourselves from what we no longer need, and keeping only what nourishes our daily lives, supports our values and reflects our essence. It's a process that's both rational and emotional.

can be confronting, but the benefits are long-lasting and profound. There are several methods for achieving this in a practical, structured and motivating way.

The KonMari method: "What brings joy".

Developed by Japanese consultant Marie Kondo, the KonMari method is based on a radically simple but profoundly transformative principle
Keep only what "brings joy". This approach, at the crossroads of minimalism and mindfulness, involves taking each object in your hands and asking yourself the following question: "Does this object spark a spark of joy in me? The answer must be immediate, visceral, almost instinctive.

What distinguishes the KonMari method from other tidying techniques is its categorical approach. Rather than sorting by room (which encourages forgetfulness), we proceed by category in a precise order:

1. Clothes
2. Books
3. Papers
4. Miscellaneous items (komono)
5. Sentimental items

Each category is dealt with in a single session, to maximise awareness. For example, gathering all your clothes in a single pile on a bed allows you to confront the extent of what you own. This makes it easier to let go, make honest choices and free up space.

This process is also emotional: we thank each object we part with for its past usefulness. This ritual, far from being anecdotal, helps to develop a healthy relationship with objects and to get rid of the guilt associated with possession.

Key point: this method is ideal for those who want to make a big sorting-out once and for all, with a strong introspective dimension. It is particularly effective for people who are sensitive, creative or seeking personal transformation.

The 90/90 rule: The test of time

Proposed by American minimalists Joshua Fields Millburn and Ryan Nicodemus, this rule is for those who prefer a functional approach, without excessive emotional involvement. It is based on two simple but powerful questions:

1. Have I used this object in the last 90 days?
2. Do I plan to use it in the next 90 days?

If the answer is no to both questions, the object is considered to be useless in your current life. The aim of this rule is to eliminate obsolete possessions, those that we keep 'just in case' but which end up weighing unnecessarily on our space and our mind.

This approach is very useful for sorting through :

- Seasonal clothes
- Kitchen tools
- Electronic items and cables
- Sports equipment
- Leisure accessories

By applying this rule to each drawer, cupboard and shelf, we can drastically simplify our environment while remaining focused on the real use. This encourages a utilitarian and pragmatic relationship with objects, without falling into emotional attachment.

Tip: create a checklist by category and systematically note down the objects that pass the test. This will also enable you to track your progress over the weeks.

The 12/12/12 method: Structure the sorting into 3 axes

If sorting seems too vague or discouraging, the 12/12/12 method is an excellent starting point. It involves identifying, during each decluttering session :

- 12 items to be thrown away (broken, out of date, unusable)
- 12 items to give away or sell
- 12 items to put away (out of place, scattered, forgotten)

This structured framework allows you to take action quickly, without asking yourself too many existential questions. It is particularly recommended for families, as it can be transformed into a collective game or challenge. For example, each member of the household can fill in their "12/12/12" and share their findings. This creates a team dynamic around simplification.

This method also helps people to become aware of their cluttering habits, by revealing where they are accumulating things unnecessarily. With repetition, it establishes a gentle, regular discipline, perfect for minimalist home maintenance.

The 30-Day Minimalist Challenge: A gradual transformation

The Minimalist Challenge is a month-long game, ideal for creating a powerful momentum for change. The principle is simple:

- Day 1: part with one object
- Day 2: two objects

- Day 3: three objects...

Until day 30, when 30 items are disposed of. In total, 465 items leave your life in 30 days.

This challenge works wonders because it creates a cumulative momentum effect: the further you go, the greater your mental clarity, motivation and sense of lightness. It also reveals the extent to which we accumulate unnecessary things without realising it. Many people finish this challenge with the feeling of having regained control over their home... and over themselves.

Tip: document the experience with before-and-after photos, or keep a diary.
logbook. This will reinforce your commitment.

The quarantine box

Some objects are difficult to dispose of straight away. Whether it's a gift, a souvenir or a potentially useful object, you may hesitate. That's where the quarantine box comes in. Simply place the object in a closed box, with a dated label, and return to it in 30, 60 or 90 days. If, when you open the box, you haven't thought about the item or needed to use it, then you don't really miss it.

This approach reduces the stress associated with sorting, because it gives you time to test your detachment, without making any immediate decisions. It's ideal for people who are new to minimalism or who feel very guilty about the idea of throwing things away.

The no duplication rule: one use, one object

Another strategy is to eliminate unnecessary duplication. We often tend to accumulate several copies of the same type of object:

- 5 pens when we only use one
- 4 chargers for a single device
- 3 identical saucepans
- Dozens of orphan socks...

Applying this rule means asking yourself the question: "Do I need several copies of this object in my day-to-day life?

In most cases, one is enough. By eliminating duplicates, you can reduce clutter, simplify storage and save precious time in your day-to-day life.

The lasting benefits of a clutter-free space

An uncluttered environment not only transforms your space, it also has a profound effect on your inner state:

- Mental clarity: fewer visual distractions = greater concentration and calm.
- Less stress: every unnecessary object is an unconscious micro-tension.
- Greater productivity: a well-organised space boosts efficiency.
- Save energy: less cleaning, sorting and maintenance.
- Spiritual awakening: decluttering also means learning to detach oneself from to refocus on what's essential.

Decluttering: a lifestyle, not an event

It's important to understand that decluttering is not a one-off task. It's a cyclical process, a mental and material lifestyle. It's about making decluttering part of your daily routine, reviewing your shopping habits, consuming with intention and valuing the essentials.

By incorporating one or more of these methods into your routine, you're not just tidying up your home: you're transforming your relationship with the world. You learn to say no to the superfluous, to make room for what really matters, and to make your space a faithful reflection of your inner life.

Organising a minimalist home: room by room

Decluttering your living space is not a one-off action, but a conscious and gradual process aimed at aligning your environment with your true needs. In a society where over-consumption is the norm, every room in the house becomes, over time, a sanctuary for the superfluous. The minimalist approach aims to reverse this trend, bringing clear structure, visual peace and enhanced functionality to every corner of the home. Working room by room is the most effective way of avoiding decision fatigue, maintaining motivation and measuring progress in concrete terms. It's a form of space therapy which, by eliminating excess, allows you to rediscover the full value of everything and reconnect with what's essential.

1. The living room: creating a space for mental breathing

The living room, often considered the heart of the home, is where the energies of all the members of the household come together. It's a place to relax, t o entertain, but also to express yourself. Yet it is often overrun by an accumulation of decorative objects, knick-knacks brought back from trips, piled-up magazines, visible cables, duplicate pieces of furniture, toys and electronic accessories.

Adopting a minimalist approach in the living room means first of all identifying what is really being used: is the sofa comfortable or just decorative? Is the coffee table useful or just imposing? Do you really need five cushions in different colours, or are two enough to create a warm atmosphere? Removing non-essential items allows the space to breathe naturally again, and calms the mind.

It is also essential to create bright areas: a reading corner with an armchair and a soft lamp, a shelf with carefully chosen books, a purifying green plant. The living room then becomes a sensory refuge, a place to welcome yourself and others, rather than a space of visual aggression.

2. The kitchen: a laboratory of simplicity

The kitchen is one of the most saturated areas of the home, often cluttered with gadgets, unused utensils, excess crockery and forgotten appliances. Minimalism, here, must rhyme with efficiency and clarity. It's not about sacrificing functionality, but optimising it by streamlining.

Start by emptying all the cupboards and sorting each item into three categories: everyday, occasional and superfluous. Ask yourself: "Do I use this item at least once a month? If the answer is no, it's time to part with it or give it away.

The aim is to keep only what's necessary: a few good quality saucepans, a set of sharp knives, a chopping board and two or three multi-purpose utensils. Limit crockery to the bare essentials. A minimalist kitchen makes meal preparation easier, cleaning quicker and reduces the mental workload associated with choosing.

Worktops should be kept clear to embody a promise of simplicity: this emptiness is not an absence, but an invitation to creation, to serenity, to full presence in everyday gestures.

3. The bedroom: a sanctuary of calm

The bedroom is much more than a place to sleep: it's an intimate, sacred space where you recharge your batteries, dream, find yourself. Yet it is often transformed into an overcrowded dressing room, a multimedia room or a makeshift office. Minimalism invites us to restore the room to its original purpose: rest.

Start by clearing your visual space. Remove anything that is not related to sleep or relaxation: television, computer equipment, decorative objects that are too stimulating, an accumulation of useless cushions. The environment should inspire calm, gentleness and letting go.

Opt for quality, uncluttered bedding in natural or sober tones. One well-organised piece of storage furniture is better than a pile of chests of drawers. Also think about reducing your wardrobe: a selection of clothes that you like, that fit, and that you wear regularly will save you the stress of making an unnecessary choice every morning.

Finally, incorporate elements that encourage deep sleep: blackout curtains, subdued lighting, soothing perfume, and above all... the visual silence of an uncluttered space.

4. The bathroom: purity and functionality

The bathroom should embody cleanliness, lightness and clarity. However, with dozens of open bottles, excess towels and forgotten beauty accessories, it quickly becomes a place of anxiety-inducing clutter. Minimalism here aims to simplify your routine and promote physical and mental hygiene.

Keep only the essentials for your daily routine. A single shampoo, neutral soap, moisturiser and deodorant. Avoid redundancy: no need for three types of scrub or four fragrances. Each product should have a clear purpose and a justified frequency of use.

Store items in closed compartments to maintain a visually clean appearance. Towels should be few in number but of good quality, folded with care. A clean mirror, soft lighting and an uncluttered floor are all micro-details that promote a feeling of freshness and control.

A minimalist bathroom makes washing pleasant, quick and almost meditative.

5. The office or work area: a bastion of mental clarity

The workspace is a direct reflection of our inner state. A cluttered desk, saturated with papers, pens, cables and post-its, becomes the scene of stress, procrastination and mental dispersion. Minimalism in the office consists of eradicating accessories to allow concentration to emerge.

Start by emptying the entire surface of the desk. Then reintroduce, one by one, the items you need for your main activity: a computer, a notebook, a pen, a lamp. Nothing else. Everything else (archived files, secondary electronic accessories) should be put away, filed or digitised.

Adopt digital document management: scan your important papers and file them in named folders. Less paper means less stress, less searching, less dust. Keep your desk clear at the end of the day at the end of the day to maintain mental hygiene and establish a clear boundary between work and relaxation.

6. The entrance: the gateway to your state of mind

The entrance to the home is often neglected, even though it gives the first impression and acts as an energy barrier between the outside world and the space inside. Well-thought-out minimalism starts here, with the elimination of anything that creates chaos: piled-up shoes, forgotten bags, unopened mail, misplaced keys.

Focus on dedicated storage: a pocket for keys, a basket for mail to be dealt with, a closed shoe cabinet. If the space is small, opt for wall-mounted solutions. The aim is to create a smooth, soothing transition between inside and outside.

You may want to add a symbolic touch: a green plant, a family photo or an inspirational phrase. The entrance then becomes an inner doorway, a reminder that at home you're getting back to basics.

7. Secondary spaces: garages, utility rooms, storage rooms

These areas are often the emotional dumping grounds of the home, where we pile up "what we don't know where to put" or "what we keep just in case". Yet a tidy garage, functional utility room or uncluttered attic can significantly improve quality of life.

Minimalism in this case calls for extra rigour. Make a drastic selection: if an object hasn't been used for a year, it can go. Tools, old clothes, unfamiliar cables, broken objects, dusty souvenirs... everything needs to be confronted with the reality of its usefulness. Everything that is kept must have a clear place, a precise function and an anticipated use.

Once uncluttered, these spaces can become secondary resources: a creative workshop, a meditation room, a space for sport or music.

Organising a minimalist home room by room means rebuilding a peaceful relationship with the space, the objects and yourself. It's an approach that goes beyond simple tidying: it touches on our way of life, our relationship with time, with need, with attachment, with emptiness. Every room becomes an exercise in introspection, every object a decision, every tidy-up an act of presence.

This process will make you more aware, lighter and freer. You won't just have a cleaner house, but a life that's clearer, more fluid, more full of meaning.

The importance of empty space

In a society dominated by hyperstimulation, over-consumption and the constant need to fill, empty space seems like an anomaly. It disturbs. It raises questions. It frightens. And yet, in the minimalist philosophy, it is one of the most fundamental pillars. Empty space is not a lack to be filled, but a conscious choice, an act of spatial and emotional intelligence. It embodies a desire to make space, not just in our homes, but also in our minds, in our schedules and, by extension, in our entire lives.

1. Emptiness as cognitive rest

Every object in our field of vision captures a fragment of our attention. Even without direct interaction, every knick-knack on a shelf, every stack of books, every piece of furniture, every piece of paper, subconsciously requires our brain to identify, interpret and categorise it. This may seem trivial, but on a daily scale day, it consumes a considerable amount of mental energy. In an overloaded environment, our minds never get a break from seeing. It's constantly in demand, even when we think we're at rest. This can generate a subtle form of latent stress, a permanent inner turmoil.

Conversely, an empty space acts like a bath of visual silence. It creates breath. It allows the eye to rest, the mind to slow down. It sends out a powerful signal: "here you can relax, you have nothing to manage, nothing to control". Emptiness frees up mental bandwidth. It gives our mind space to refocus, to process its own thoughts without outside distraction. In this way, emptiness is a form of mental hygiene, an environment that allows us to be fully with ourselves, without interference.

2. Emptiness as a revelation of the essential

In a saturated space, everything loses its importance. The eye no longer knows where to land. It glides from one object to another without ever lingering. What should have value - a souvenir, a painting, an object of art - drowns in the mass. Emptiness, on the other hand, acts as an enhancing frame. It surrounds, it highlights, i t prioritises. It gives weight to what is present. It transforms a simple object into a focal point. It draws attention to what really deserves to be seen, admired or used.

It's the same principle as in a museum: the works are not piled up, they are spaced out, highlighted by the emptiness around them. In our homes, exactly the same thing happens. By simplifying our space, by deliberately leaving certain surfaces clear - a table without objects, a wall without decoration, a piece of furniture with just one item on it - we allow everything present to exist fully. We reconnect with its function, its beauty, its meaning.

3. Emptiness as an emotional and spiritual anchor

This is not just an aesthetic or practical issue. Emptiness also has a profoundly emotional, even spiritual dimension. It represents an opening. It is the space through which peace, clarity, creativity and presence can enter. In many spiritual traditions, emptiness is sacred. It is the place of inner silence, the point of access to intuition, meditation, connection with oneself or with a greater dimension.

When you empty your material space, you're doing more than just tidying up: you're symbolically ridding yourself of the things that clutter up your soul. Every object you remove is one less mental attachment. A commitment, a memory, an implicit obligation to "do something with it". By leaving a vacuum in our environment, we create an inner climate conducive to introspection, lightness and detachment. We rediscover the pleasure of living in a place that doesn't suffocate us, but welcomes us.

4. Emptiness as a refocusing tool

Empty space is also a formidable tool for existential clarity. In a world that constantly pushes us to accumulate objects, relationships, activities and information, emptiness is a gentle but radical form of resistance. It says: "I choose not to disperse myself". It affirms an intention to refocus, a desire to keep only what is consistent with our values, our needs and our projects. Each void created is an act of sorting, prioritising.

For example, leaving a wall empty means refusing the injunction to decorate systematically. Keeping space in a library means recognising that we don't have to read everything, own everything or display everything. Leaving space in a room means giving yourself the right to move, to dance, to breathe, to live without constraints. In this way, the void becomes an invisible structure that supports our freedom, rather than enclosing it.

5. The void as a space for transformation

Finally, it is essential to understand that the void is alive. It is not frozen. It is not a void, but a potential in the making. It opens a door. It allows change. Where everything is already full, nothing can enter. Nothing can evolve. By creating emptiness, we free up space for the new: a new habit, a new project, a new relationship, a new state of being.

The emptiness is a call. A call to listen to yourself. To patience. To presence. It reminds us that we don't have to fill everything right away. That lack is not necessarily a problem. That it is sometimes a fertile zone of waiting, of germination, of silent transformation. It is in the void that movement is born. It is in the void that our lives can be reinvented.

Adopting minimalism doesn't just mean owning less. It also means learning to appreciate emptiness, to respect it, to honour it. It's a counter-cultural process, often disturbing at first, but profoundly liberating. Emptiness then becomes our ally. It calms our mind, it values the essential, it opens us up to introspection, it refocuses our attention, and it welcomes future transformations. Simplifying your space means making room for the invisible, the intimate, the important. It's about giving yourself a framework in which peace can finally take hold.

Chapter 5: Digital minimalism

Managing digital overload (e-mails, social networks, notifications)

In today's hyper-connected world, human attention has become a rare and coveted resource. Every sound, vibration or red badge on a screen represents an often successful attempt to divert our concentration. Digital overload, this insidious but omnipresent phenomenon, causes continuous mental fatigue, a drop in productivity and a diffuse but persistent form of anxiety. To apply minimalism to everyday life in a practical way, it is essential to learn how to tame this overload. This process begins by rebalancing our relationship with digital tools, by returning technology to the role of assistant rather than mistress.

1. Controlling your email inbox: getting out of the trap of constant urgency

The e-mail inbox has become a place of mental confinement for millions of people. The accumulation of unread messages, constant notifications and the feeling of having to reply quickly to everything create an illusion of perpetual urgency. Yet very few emails require an immediate response, and even fewer are really important. Digital minimalism applies a fundamental principle here: conscious prioritisation.

Start by unclogging your inbox. Deleting unnecessary email isn't just an administrative task: it's a mental release. Use the "Inbox Zero" rule: your aim is to have an empty or almost empty inbox by the end of the day. Divide emails into simple categories: Reply

Today, To be read later, Archive. This avoids repetitive decisions and frees up cognitive time. Next, unsubscribe en masse from any newsletters or promotions that you haven't opened in the last three months. These messages represent digital noise, not useful information.

Finally, set yourself specific times to check your e-mails, ideally two or three times a day. Resist the temptation to leave the e-mail tab open: each new alert pulls you away from your core work and fragments your attention. Let your colleagues or friends know about your new consultation times: this creates a culture of respect for concentration time, and reduces the pressure of immediacy.

2. Tame social networks: regain control of your attention

Social networks are not intrinsically bad. They allow us to keep in touch, to keep informed and to express ourselves. The problem is the compulsive and passive use we make of them, often without even realising it. Every swipe, every like, every story feeds a loop of dopamine. These platforms exploit precise psychological mechanisms to capture and hold our attention for as long as possible. The result: hours stolen every week, attention scattered, self-esteem weakened by constant comparison.

Adopting a minimalist approach means first of all carrying out a radical audit of your relationship with the networks. How much time do you spend on them every day? Why do you open them? What do you get out of them: inspiration or frustration? Start by uninstalling the applications that don't bring you any real value. Then delete or mute accounts that make you feel inferior, frustrated or passive. Give priority to content that uplifts you, makes you think or encourages you to take action in real life.

You can also introduce a digital diet: one or two days a week without any social networks, or even a whole week every month. Take advantage of these moments to observe your mind: the urge to scroll is often just an escape from boredom or anxiety. The more you consciously resist it, the more you regain control of your inner life. Replace these moments of waiting with reading, writing, walking or silence: you'll notice a marked increase in your mental clarity, creativity and inner peace.

3. Cut out notifications: get away from the tyranny of the ping

Notifications are a modern form of sensory aggression. They demand our attention, often abruptly and unjustifiably, for information that is rarely useful. Every ping, every vibration, every pop-up causes a break in concentration, even if it only lasts a second. In the long term, this deteriorates our capacity for deep work and generates psychological fatigue that is difficult to quantify.

Start by tidying up your notification settings. Go through all your applications and ask yourself, honestly: "Do I really need to receive an alert from this application?" In 90% of cases, the answer is no. Deactivate all notifications except those that are vital (urgent calls, text messages from loved ones, reminders of important appointments). For the rest - social networks, games, promotions, commercial applications - turn everything off. Your phone should no longer bother you: it's up to you to decide when to use it.

You should also get into the habit of regularly activating the "Do not disturb" mode, particularly during work periods, at mealtimes or in the evening. Better still, set aside screen-free times of the day, particularly in the morning when you wake up and in the evening before you go to sleep. These are crucial times when the brain is programming itself. If you're bombarded with notifications as soon as you wake up, you're already delegating control of your day to outside forces.

4. Organise an uncluttered digital space: clear the clutter to breathe easier

Your digital space reflects your mental state. A computer desktop saturated with files, a smartphone full of unused applications, a browser with 27 open tabs... all these elements create visual pollution that slows down not only your machine, but also your thoughts.

Start with a digital spring clean. Delete the applications you haven't used this month. Reorganise your home screen so that only the essential tools remain. Create a clean desktop on your computer, with clearly named and prioritised folders. Close all unnecessary tabs, then install an extension like OneTab to group them together if necessary. The cleaner your space, the clearer your mind.

Also, reduce the number of digital tools you use. If you have three note apps, two diaries and four email platforms, your attention is constantly fragmented. Choose one tool for each function, and learn to use it to the full. This technological refocusing will save you a huge amount of time and give you peace of mind.

5. Developing digital mental hygiene: using technology with intention

The heart of digital minimalism lies not just in elimination, but in intentionality. It's not about giving up modern tools, but about using them in a way that's aligned with your values, your priorities and your mental well-being.

Adopt the reflex of setting a clear intention before each digital interaction. Before opening your phone or computer, ask yourself: "Why am I doing this? What do I want to achieve?" This simple question breaks the automatism and transforms your relationship with technology. Get into the habit of get into the habit of jotting down in a notebook the times when you've felt absorbed or frustrated by your digital uses: this will help you spot the triggers and get a better grip on them.

Finally, replace your digital automatisms with rewarding rituals. When you feel the need to scroll, ask yourself: is it because you're tired, stressed or bored? And instead of giving in, choose a restorative activity: drink a cup of tea in silence, listen to soothing music, do some stretching, write down how you're feeling. Little by little, you'll transform these moments of escape into moments of presence.

Managing digital overload is not just a matter of technological discipline, it's an act of personal sovereignty. It means refusing to allow your mental life to be dictated by algorithms, incessant interruptions and artificial demands. By taking back control of your email inbox, your networks, your notifications and your digital environment, you gain precious space.
of inner silence, regained concentration and psychic autonomy.
autonomy.

You don't have to be reachable at all times. You don't have to see, like or read everything. By limiting your digital exposure, you broaden your scope for real freedom. Digital minimalism, applied on a daily basis, is a path towards a denser, calmer, more present life - a life where you choose where your attention goes, and therefore, where your life goes.

Digital detox: why and how

1. Because our attention has become a consumer product

In today's economy, attention has become the most coveted resource. Digital companies, whether they're social networks, streaming platforms or mobile applications, aren't selling products: they're selling our attention time to advertisers. This means that every algorithm, every notification, every interface design is designed to do one thing: keep us connected for as long as possible. This subtle and often invisible manipulation has a profound effect on our brains. We think we use our phone by choice, but in reality much of our use is reactive, impulsive and conditioned. So a digital detox is not a fad, but an act of reclaiming our mental free will.

2. Because information overload exhausts our brains

Every day, our minds are bombarded by thousands of digital stimuli: news, messages, adverts, short videos, multiple calls for attention. The problem is not the information itself, but the frenetic pace and lack o f prioritisation. The human brain needs silence, pauses and sequential processing. Yet digital technology imposes a permanent multitasking mode that leads to a form of chronic cognitive fatigue. This saturation prevents deep thought and lasting memory, and creates a form of constant inner turmoil. A digital detox helps to slow down the flow, lighten the mind, and regain the mental clarity needed for a centred, calm life.

3. Because excessive use of screens fragments our relationships and our presence

It has become commonplace to be both physically present and psychologically absent. During a meal with friends, family or even as a couple, how often do we discreetly consult our phone? This hyper-connection distances us from others, but above all from ourselves. We experience a hidden emotional disconnection. By responding to a notification, we leave the present moment and enter a digital loop, sometimes with no immediate return. A digital detox is not just an act of mental health, it's a strong relational gesture, a way of saying to another person: "I'm here. Completely."

4. Because digital technology has a direct impact on our physical health and our sleep

The impact of digital technology is not limited to our minds. The blue light from screens disrupts the production of melatonin, which is essential for falling asleep. Compulsive telephone use in bed activates the brain when it should be decompressing. The result: trouble sleeping, morning tiredness, difficulty concentrating during the day. Added to this are postural problems (bent neck, hunched back), eye pain and migraines linked to prolonged exposure. A well-executed detox restores the body's natural resting cycle and promotes overall physical well-being.

5. Because an overloaded digital life disconnects us from our core identity deep

The more we are exposed to digital content, the more we absorb, sometimes unconsciously, standards, comparisons and injunctions. Social networks, in particular, act as showcases for idealised lives. This creates a distortion of reality that erodes self-esteem, nurtures feelings of inferiority and pushes us to live up to external expectations. The digital detox is a way of reconnecting with our inner compass. It allows us to ask this fundamental question: "What drives me, me, deep down, away from the screens?"

How do you set up an effective digital detox?

1. Define your intention clearly

A detox should not be experienced as a punishment, but as a conscious act of liberation. So start by asking yourself one simple question

Why do I need to disconnect? Is it to make more time for myself? To improve my sleep? To reconnect with my loved ones? This intention will serve as a compass during the period of disconnection. Without it, you run the risk of experiencing detox as a frustrating deprivation rather than an enriching experience.

2. Set precise but realistic rules

A successful digital detox relies on the establishment of concrete frameworks. It's not It doesn't necessarily mean cutting out everything overnight. It may involve :

- Cutting the phone after 8pm every evening;
- Deleting time-consuming applications (social networks, games) for a week;
- Avoid using the telephone in the presence of others;
- Set aside one whole day a week without screens (e.g. Sunday)
  ;
- Use a basic telephone at the weekend.

The important thing is to adjust the rules to suit your lifestyle, while remaining firm about applying them.

3. Create rewarding substitution rituals

The digital detox creates a vacuum, and this vacuum can become a source of anxiety if it is not filled. That's why you need to intentionally fill it with nourishing activities: reading, meditation, writing, walking, music, drawing, cooking, sport, deep conversations. It's not just a question of turning off the screens, but of reinvesting our time in richer experiences that are more rooted in reality.

4. Remove digital temptations at source

Willpower alone is not always enough. To achieve a successful detox, it's essential to make access to digital more difficult:

- Deactivate all non-essential notifications;
- Disconnect from your accounts;
- Put your phone in another room;
- Use blocking applications (such as Forest, Freedom, Focus);
- Temporarily delete addictive applications.

This principle is based on a simple idea: reduce the friction of making the right decision.

5. Reintegrate digital media with discernment after detoxing

A detox only makes sense if it leads to a lasting change in your relationship with digital. The aim is not to become technophobic, but to reuse technology with intention. This involves :

- Introducing limited screen time each day;
- A prioritising of uses : information communication, entertainment;

- Regular assessment of the impact of digital tools on our well-being.

In the long run, we will no longer be subjected to digital technology: we will choose it, manage it and tame it. Digital detox, a pillar of inner minimalism

A digital detox is more than just uninstalling an application or switching off your Wi-Fi. It's about refocusing our lives. It teaches us to distinguish the useful from the accessory, the real from the virtual, the essential from the superfluous. It's a process that takes courage, but offers an immense reward

It brings us back to ourselves. Fewer distractions mean more depth. Fewer screens mean more presence. Less stimulation means more peace.

Creating a calm and productive digital space

In a society where the majority of interactions, work and even leisure activities take place via digital interfaces, it's becoming vital to think about how our digital environment influences our quality of life. Screens, designed to capture our attention, have become places of mental dispersion and cognitive overload. Visual noise, constant interruptions, the fragmentation of our time and the illusion of productivity cause stress, anxiety, mental fatigue and chronic dissatisfaction. Applying minimalism to our digital space means rediscovering a healthier, more conscious and, above all, more balanced relationship with technology. It means creating a digital sanctuary, conducive to concentration, creativity and inner calm.

1. Declutter to breathe easier: sorting through digital clutter

Digital clutter acts like an invisible parasite. Dozens of installed but unused applications, hundreds of duplicate photos, documents scattered in illogical directories, an overflowing email inbox - these are all signs of silent mental overload. Digital clutter is not trivial: it unconsciously demands our attention, creating a feeling of chaos and stealing precious time.

To remedy this, start with a weekly digital decluttering session. Organise your files into simple, clear categories: "Administrative documents", "Current projects", "Archives", "To be sorted". Delete obsolete files, duplicates and irrelevant notes, and create a logical structure in your folders. Your computer desktop should not become a graveyard of temporary files. Ideally, it should remain empty or contain only a few essential shortcuts, as a sober gateway to your digital universe.

Apply the same sorting process to your mobile devices. Delete all the applications you haven't used in the last month. Ask yourself a simple but powerful question: "Does this app serve my values, priorities or goals?" If the answer is no, it doesn't belong on your screen.

2. Eliminate distractions: control notifications and constant interruption

Notifications have become the new shackles of the modern mind. Every sound alert, vibration or red badge is an attempt to capture our attention. They are constant intrusions into our mental field, fragmenting our concentration, reducing our ability to enter a state of 'flow' (deep concentration), and conditioning us to reactivity rather than concentration.

of deep concentration), and condition us to reactivity rather than intention.

To create a serene digital environment, you need to restore a form of sovereignty over your attention. Start by carrying out a complete audit of your notification settings. On your phone, deactivate all non-essential notifications. This includes social networks, online shops, news, and even certain promotional messages from banking or transport applications. Keep only what's vital: calls, messages from friends and family, reminders of important appointments.

Go further by activating "Do Not Disturb" modes during deep work or rest periods. Define precise periods during the day (for example, from 9am to 11am, or from 8pm to 10pm) when no device should interrupt what you're doing. In addition, limit the number of times you check your email inboxes or social networks. Establish checking routines (for example, three times a day: morning, midday and late afternoon), and stick to them. In this way, you'll regain control over the tempo of your mental life.

3. Clean up the aesthetics: lighten the visual environment

The visual environment of your interfaces has a direct impact on your mental state. Cluttered icons, busy wallpapers, gaudy colours and applications with complex interfaces increase the cognitive load, distract the eye and generate stress without you being aware of it. Digital minimalism therefore also involves a pure, soothing design.

Opt for a sober screen background in neutral or natural tones. A photo of a soothing landscape, a soft abstract image, or simply a solid colour can be enough to create a calm effect. Organise your icons according to logical function, by theme or by frequency of use, and avoid duplication. On your smartphone, try to reduce the number of screens to one by creating organised folders. Place essential applications within easy reach and relegate those that deliberately distract you to a less accessible location, or even hide them.

Digital design should reflect your desire for clarity. Less visual clutter means more mental lightness. When you open your phone or computer, you shouldn't feel like you're entering a battlefield of tabs, but a clear, fluid, functional space.

4. Structure your digital day: adopt conscious digital rituals

Creating a calm digital space depends not just on what you see, but on when and how you use your tools. Without structure, digital invades every corner of your day, like water seeping in everywhere. The key here is to ritualise your use.

Start by establishing a screen-free morning routine. Set aside the first 30 to 60 minutes of your day for offline activities: drinking a glass of mindful water, writing in a journal, meditating, walking outside or reading a paper book. This sends a clear message to your brain: "I'm in control of the tempo o f my day." Avoid the reflex of immediately consulting your phone when you wake up: this immediately puts you in a reactive posture, often tinged with stress.

Continue with a structured digital timetable. Define the times when you check your email from 10am to 10.30am, social networks from 1pm to 1.15pm and news from 6pm to 6.20pm. Outside these times, the platforms concerned remain closed. This rigour may seem austere at first, but it becomes a liberating discipline in the long run.

Finally, consider incorporating a digital closing routine in the evening. An hour before bedtime, step away from the screens, reduce the blue light, and engage in a relaxing activity. This simple habit will improve the quality of your sleep and protect your nervous system from unnecessary stimuli.

5. Rethinking our relationship with technology: cultivating intentional use

Digital minimalism is not a fad, but a philosophy of life. It's not about rejecting technology, but about redefining our relationship with it. Instead of being subjected to digital tools, we need to use them as conscious extensions of our will.

The central question is: "Am I using this technology, or is it using me? This awareness radically transforms the way we use it. You can replace moments of digital emptiness (passive scrolling, constant zapping) with intentional practices: reading an article in depth, taking a training course, writing down your thoughts, or creating content that reflects you.

Reducing the number of platforms on which you are active, refusing useless social notifications and stopping replying immediately to every message are acts of reappropriation. You're no longer escaping into the digital world. You consciously inhabit it. You are no longer a product, but a player.

Creating a calm and productive digital space is not a luxury option, but a necessity for mental health in today's world. It means giving yourself the means to think clearly, feel deeply, create freely and live fully. By applying the principles of digital minimalism, you transform every interaction with technology into an act of mindfulness. You choose quality over quantity, intention over compulsion, presence over distraction.

Your digital space then becomes a faithful reflection of your inner space: clear, aligned and deeply human.

Chapter 6: Minimalism in finance

Rethinking your consumption

Minimalism applied to finance cannot be fully effective without a profound change in our relationship to consumption. We live in an age when the act of buying is no longer merely functional, but has become emotional, impulsive, almost identity-related. We consume to feel we exist, to reward ourselves, to fill a void or to resemble an ideal image that we are sold through social networks and advertising. But rethinking our consumption means deconstructing this logic. It means undergoing a mental and behavioural revolution: we no longer consume out of habit or to follow an external norm, but with intention, awareness and personal alignment.

Distinguishing between needs, desires and impulses

The first step in rethinking our consumption is to get back to basics: understanding the difference between a need, a want and an impulse. A need is an objective necessity (food, shelter, clothing for protection). A craving, on the other hand, is a subjective desire, often influenced b y emotional or social factors. An impulse, on the other hand, is the result of a quick, thoughtless reaction to an external stimulus (lightning promotion, targeted advertising, fashion effect).

All too often, our finances suffer because we let these impulses guide our buying decisions. How many items of clothing lie dormant in our wardrobes, bought because "it was a good deal"? How many technological items have become obsolete as soon as they were unpacked? Minimalism invites us to be clear-headed: does this purchase bring me real value in the long term? Does it improve my life? Does it meet a need or an illusion?

?

Cultivate patience before each purchase

In a society of immediacy, where everything is just a click away, delaying the act of buying is a radically minimalist gesture. A simple but powerful strategy is to allow yourself 48 to 72 hours to think about any non-essential expenditure. This period acts as a natural filter: if the urge persists after this time, it may be a worthwhile purchase; if it has evaporated, it was merely a passing impulse.

By taking a step back, you can regain power over the emotional marketing that pushes you to consume in a hurry: "Limited offer", "Only 2 left in stock", "End in 3 hours". By taking a step back, we can transform compulsive consumption i n t o thoughtful, responsible consumption, in line with our financial objectives and our mental well-being.

De-programming over-consumption reflexes

Rethinking our consumption requires us to work on deprogramming our minds. Since childhood, we have been conditioned to associate buying with reward, success and recognition. Minimalism invites us to break with this conditioning by identifying the unconscious patterns that dictate our buying behaviour. This can involve :

- A complete audit of our spending habits (where does the money go? which purchases are recurrent but not very useful?

  (Where does the money go? Which purchases are recurrent but not very useful?)

- Becoming aware of emotional triggers (do I buy when I'm bored?

  when I'm bored, when I feel bad, to compensate for stress).

- Reflecting on the symbolic needs linked to consumption (buying to be loved, to impress, to feel like you exist).

By understanding that we don't need to "own more" to be "more", we begin a mental detox from consumerism as a solution to our emotions or insecurities.

Reorienting value: quality, utility, sustainability

Minimalism is not a call for deprivation, but a call for intelligent selection. This means prioritising quality over quantity, real utility over appearance, durability over fleeting novelty. A well-tailored, durable, versatile garment is better than five cheap items that will only be worn once. A reliable, eco-designed, repairable household appliance is better than a state-of-the-art but fragile gadget.

Rethinking our consumption also means taking into account the total cost of ownership: beyond the purchase price, how much will this object cost to maintain, repair and replace? Will it make my life easier or more cumbersome? By developing this overall awareness of the impact of a purchase, we consume less, but better, and our finances naturally become healthier.

Adopt a logic of circularity

Minimalism also encourages circular consumption: reuse, repair, recycle, barter. This approach, far from being marginal, is now facilitated by numerous platforms (Vinted, Leboncoin, Geev, Emmaüs). It allows you to

Not only can you save money, but you can also reduce your ecological footprint and clear up clutter.

For example:

- Before buying something new, ask yourself: can I borrow or hire it?
- Before throwing something away, ask yourself: can I repair it, transform it or give it away?
- Before storing, think: am I still using it? If not, can I sell it?

This more circular way of consuming transforms our daily lives into a fluid ecosystem, where objects circulate, find a second life, and don't become financial or mental burdens.

Freeing up mental and financial capital

As we consume less and consume better, a natural consequence occurs: we spend less money, of course, but we also gain mental peace of mind. Every purchase you avoid means one less mental burden: no need to tidy it up, maintain it or keep an eye on it. Less clutter means more clarity of mind.

These savings can be used strategically: precautionary savings, investment, financing a meaningful project (travel, retraining, education). It's no longer money that's diluted in a thousand micro-spendings, but financial energy refocused on what really matters to you.

Consuming in line with your values

Finally, rethinking our consumption means making every expenditure an act of personal consistency. Instead of giving in to the temptation of immediate gratification

Instead of giving in to the temptation of immediate gratification, we ask ourselves: does this reflect my convictions? Does it respect my ecological, social and human principles? Does it help me to become the person I want to be?

By choosing to support ethical, local and transparent brands, or by refusing to feed destructive industries, we regain ethical control over our purchasing power. We transform consumption into a conscious, militant and responsible act in the service of a fairer world and a more aligned life.

Living below your means

A paradigm shift in the face of a consumer society

Living within your means is more than just a budgeting exercise; it's a philosophy of life, a real reversal of the norms imposed by modern society. For decades, advertising, social networks, fashion and popular culture have conditioned us to associate happiness with consumption. Own, display, renew, accumulate: these silent injunctions form a constant background noise. And without realising it, we become dependent on a rhythm of life dictated by our spending.

Financial minimalism breaks this cycle. It invites us to stop spending to fill emotional gaps or meet external standards, and to align our finances with our deepest values. Living below your means is not about restricting yourself for the sake of deprivation; it's about deliberately choosing not to spend every euro you earn, in order to regain control o f your future.

Distinguishing between apparent wealth and real security

Many people have a high standard of living but fragile finances. They earn a good living, but sometimes spend more. The result: no savings, outstanding consumer credit and a constant fear of the unexpected. This is a common paradox: people who are financially "well off" are in fact living in permanent instability.

Conversely, those who live below their means may have a modest income but enjoy a rare peace of mind. Because true wealth lies not in what you show, but in what you keep. It is measured by the ability to deal with the unexpected, to say no to a toxic job, to take well-considered risks, to invest in meaningful projects.

This lifestyle creates a financial buffer zone: a margin between what you earn and what you spend. And this margin is precious. It acts as a bumper against the vagaries of life (breakdown, accident, job loss) and becomes a strategic tool for building a life that is intentional, free and resilient.

Rethink your needs with clarity

Living below your means means reconsidering your needs. It starts with honest introspection: "What do I really need to live well? We often realise that many of our expenses are linked to automatisms, passing desires or social pressures. For example:

- Do I really need a premium subscription to all the streaming p l a t f o r m s ?
- Is it essential to change your phone every year?

- Are expensive weekend outings a necessity or an empty routine?
- Is buying clothes every month a real need or a strategy to fill an emotional void?

Minimalism encourages us to sort out the necessary, the useful and the superficial. It encourages us to consume consciously, to ask ourselves questions before each expenditure, to stop looking for immediate gratification and to build lasting satisfaction.

Revaluing sobriety as an engine of power

In popular culture, sobriety has long been associated with poverty or lack. But in a minimalist vision, sobriety is an act of power. It means: "I choose what goes into my life. I am no longer a slave to my desires. I control my impulses. I'm building my freedom".

Living within your means means that you :

- Not be dependent on credit or outside help
- Refuse jobs or projects that run counter to your values
- Save for the future or invest in your passions
- Travel or take time off without financial anxiety
- Build a sustainable, stable, aligned life

This chosen sobriety makes you freer, more confident and more serene. It restores its rightful place: as a tool, not a master.

Curbing lifestyle inflation: the silent trap

One of the most insidious traps preventing people from living below their means is lifestyle inflation. This is the mechanism by which, as soon as income rises, expenditure follows or even exceeds it. Y o u start living in more expensive accommodation, buying designer clothes, eating out more often and going on holiday further afield.

The result is a feeling of always being on the verge of overdraft, even on a good salary. This never-ending race prevents you from capitalising on your efforts. Financial minimalism offers a radical alternative: voluntarily stabilise your lifestyle even if you earn more. This allows you to turn every increase in income into savings, investments or opportunities.

This is how silent fortunes are born. Not the ones that show off, but the ones that are built in the shadows, thanks to an invisible but powerful financial discipline.

Create a minimalist budget in line with your priorities

If you really want to live within your means, it's essential to budget intelligently. Minimalism doesn't reject the budget - on the contrary, it simplifies it. The aim is to reduce secondary items of expenditure and optimise those that really count.

You can use simple rules such as :

- The 50/30/20 rule: 50% for needs, 30% for desires, 20% for savings or investment.
  for savings or investment
- The "pay yourself first" rule: save as soon as the income comes in, before any expenditure.
  any expenditure
- The "zero base" method: allocate every euro to a task (even if the
  savings are planned)

The aim is not deprivation, but intentionality: every euro spent must correspond to a conscious choice. A minimalist budget is a tool for aligning your finances, your life goals and your values.

Investing the difference: transforming sobriety into a lever for wealth

What differentiates a minimalist from someone who is simply thrifty is what they do with the money they don't spend. They don't just save it, they invest it strategically. This can include:

- Build up an emergency fund equivalent to 3 to 6 months' expenditure
- Invest in ETFs (low-cost stock market indices)
- Buy shares in SCPIs to generate passive property income
- Take a training course to develop a monetisable skill
- Launch an entrepreneurial project with impact

Every euro not spent becomes a seed sown for the future. This is how sobriety becomes growth, how today's simplicity becomes tomorrow's wealth.

Invest in what really matters

In a world where our attention is constantly captured by advertising, social networks and consumer trends, it can be difficult to distinguish between our real needs and our fleeting desires. Yet this is precisely where financial minimalism finds all its strength: it suggests that we slow down, question ourselves, and consciously redirect our money towards what truly enriches our lives. Investing in what really matters means learning to consciously choose how we use our resources, in order to

align our financial reality with our deepest values, and not with external
external pressures.

1. Understanding what really matters: the clarity exercise

Before we even talk about money, we need to ask ourselves what direction we want
our lives to take. This starts with introspection: what really makes you happy? What
gives you a sense of meaning, fulfilment and inner peace? For some, it might be the
freedom to travel or to work for yourself. For others, it might be health, the safety of
loved ones, or access to culture, nature or personal development.

Once these values have been identified, they become a financial compass. Any
investment or expenditure must pass through the filter of this compass. Does what I'm
about to buy really contribute to a richer, more aligned, more serene life? Does it
nourish what is essential to me, or is it   a   distraction   costly   which
takes me away   from   myself   ? With this clarity, we can already eliminate
hundreds of unnecessary purchases, false needs and automatic consumer habits.

2. Reducing parasitic expenditure to free up resources

Minimalism does not advocate austerity, but the elimination of waste. And this waste
is omnipresent: forgotten subscriptions, items bought on the spur of the moment and
never used, unjustified bank charges, double clothing, superfluous electronic
equipment... All these expenses parasitise our mental space as much as our budget.

Every expense avoided becomes an available resource: not only financially, but also
in terms of energy. Because the less we consume, the less

the less we maintain, the less we manage. And this gain in mental energy is considerable. This energy can then be channelled into what deeply nourishes us: a passion, a project, training, investing in our health, or spending time with loved ones.

This refocusing teaches us a simple but powerful truth: every euro spent is a vote. It's a vote for the lifestyle we build, for the kind of person we become. And that makes every purchase choice infinitely more important than its mere monetary value.

3. Spend less to invest better

By reallocating money not spent unnecessarily, you can start to invest intelligently, even with small sums. The idea is not to become rich quickly, but to build a sustainable, stable situation that b r i n g s us freedom.

A minimalist budget is not a fixed budget. It's a living, dynamic budget that serves as a springboard for long-term projects. It could be :

- A training course leading to a qualification that will enable you to retrain for a job that is more in line with your values.
- Simple financial investments in ETFs or SCPIs that generate passive income over the long term.
- A memorable trip, a silent retreat, or a personal development p r o g r a m m e that transforms you.
- The purchase o f a modest but healthy home that frees you from rental stress and anchors you.
- Or investing in your health: specialist consultations, quality food, adapted sport, restful sleep...

In this way, money becomes a tool for freedom rather than an object of accumulation or social status.

4. Distinguish between genuine investments and disguised expenditure

A common mistake is to believe that certain expenses are investments, when in fact they are not. Buying the latest smartphone every year "to work faster", buying a luxury car "to make a good impression", or regularly changing your interior decoration to "feel good at home": these are often expenses disguised as investments, but which in reality meet needs for appearance or instant emotion.

The real investment is the one that has a return over time: a financial return, a return in freedom, a return in energy, or a return in knowledge. It makes your life easier, more stable and more fluid over time. It has a clear, measurable intention, and above all it is part of a long-term vision.

Adopting this rigour requires a paradigm shift: from reactive consumerism to conscious mastery. It's not easy at first, as it often involves resisting social norms. But in the long run, this posture creates a lighter, more coherent life that is richer inside.

5. Create a minimalist investment routine

Investing in what really matters is not a one-off act, it's a daily discipline. This means setting up a clear, stable and adjustable routine:

- Every month, allocate a fixed percentage of your income to selected investments (training, savings, stock portfolio, donations, etc.).

- Regularly re-evaluate what is really useful, and adjust your choices choices accordingly.
- Monitor your budget not to restrict yourself, but to measure your drift and progress.
- Get into the habit of deferring purchases for 48 hours or a week, so that you only keep only what you really want.
- Keep a financial gratitude diary: note down what you already own, what you've invested, and how it improves your life.

This system promotes lasting inner peace. You stop chasing after more and start appreciating more. You enjoy simplicity and marvel at the freedom it brings.

Investing in what really matters means choosing a life that's aligned rather than one that's full. It means understanding that money is not an end, but a means of building a life that is richer inside, freer and more serene. It means refusing to live according to imposed models, and instead creating a path that makes sense - a path that is sober, elegant and clear.

Financial minimalism is not a savings technique. It's a philosophy of life. And every time you invest in what really matters, you stop buying distractions and become the author of your own life.

Chapter 7: Relationship minimalism

Quality rather than quantity in relationships

One of the most transformative aspects of minimalism applied to everyday life concerns our relationships. More than just a way of clearing away material clutter, relational minimalism encourages us to re-evaluate the place we give to human relationships in our lives, not in terms of numbers, but in terms of depth, appropriateness and sincerity. In an age where over-connection reigns and we often accumulate dozens, even hundreds of contacts on social networks, it becomes crucial to ask ourselves: do I really feel surrounded or simply overloaded? Do these relationships nourish me... or exhaust me?

?

1. The illusion of relationship abundance

The modern world values hyper-socialisation. Having a large network of friends, being in constant demand, appearing sociable and surrounded are all perceived as signs of social success. Yet this apparent abundance often masks a great superficiality. Increasing the number of connections can become a flight into danger: fear of being alone, need for recognition, fear of missing out. So we maintain superficial connections, where we talk a lot but say nothing of substance. We spread ourselves too thin, forcing ourselves to maintain relationships out of convention, politeness or habit, to the detriment of ourselves. Relational minimalism invites us to get away from this illusion and recognise that it's not the number of people around us that determines our happiness in relationships, but the quality of the interactions we experience.

2. The emotional fatigue of unaligned relationships

Every relationship, however light, mobilises a part of our mental and emotional energy. Responding to messages, accepting invitations out of obligation, listening to other people's problems without reciprocating, maintaining links that no longer resonate with our innermost being... all this constitutes an invisible but real burden. Over time, these unaligned relationships become a source of emotional fatigue, discomfort and even frustration. Minimalism in relationships means making a clear distinction: not out of contempt or rejection, but out of self-respect. It means asking yourself concrete questions: "Does this person pull me up? "Can I be myself in their presence? "Does this relationship bring me peace or stress? This work of conscious selection is not a selfish act, but an act of responsibility towards our inner balance.

3. The transformative power of authentic relationships

When we voluntarily reduce the number of relationships we have and concentrate on a few sincere and deep ones, a powerful phenomenon occurs: these relationships become truer, more nourishing and more stable. You stop playing a role, trying to please or meet external expectations. We enter a dimension where the exchange becomes truly human: active listening, honest speech, shared vulnerability. In a small circle, everyone has their place. You no longer need to be seen by everyone, because you are seen in depth by just a few. These relationships become solid anchors, refuges in stormy waters, sources of lasting joy. By choosing quality, we create a social life that is less noisy, but infinitely richer.

4. The art of saying no: setting limits without guilt

Reducing the number of relationships we have often means having to say no: no t o solicitations, to unbalanced friendships, to toxic relationship dynamics. This takes courage, because we have often been conditioned to please, to avoid conflict, to maintain relationships even when they no longer suit us. Yet learning to say no, respectfully but firmly, is essential to a minimalist approach. Saying no to the outside world means saying yes to yourself. It means setting clear limits to preserve your energy, mental peace and emotional freedom. Minimalism in relationships teaches that any lasting relationship is based on a balance between giving and receiving, between opening up and protecting your inner space.

5. Welcoming solitude as a fertile space

When you reduce your network of contacts, it's natural to go through phases of loneliness. But contrary to widespread belief, solitude is not a void to be filled, but a fertile space to be inhabited. It allows us to reconnect with ourselves, rediscover our deepest desires, explore our creativity and listen to our intuition. This time without superficial interactions becomes a time of regeneration. We learn to be self-sufficient, no longer constantly dependent on external approval to feel we exist. As a result, the relationships we choose afterwards are no longer motivated by lack or fear, but by a desire for sincere, reciprocal exchange.

6. Building a relationship ecosystem in line with your life vision

Finally, relationship minimalism is not about isolation, but about rebuilding. It's about creating a relationship ecosystem that is consistent with your values, aspirations and vision of the world. Sometimes this means leaving old social circles to join new, more inspiring ones that are closer to your current inner vibrations. This can mean opening up to inter-generational relationships, getting closer to people who share the same spiritual quest or passion, or simply moving away from old social circles.

or passion, or simply deepening family ties with sincere loved ones. This new, smaller but more solid circle becomes a stable base from which to develop fully, without dispersion, pretense or chronic social fatigue.

By applying the principle of quality rather than quantity in relationships, relational minimalism gives us back power over our inner world. It frees us from invisible constraints, makes us more present in our exchanges, and transforms human relationships into what they should always be: a place of reciprocity, truth and mutual evolution. Choosing our relationships is not about closing ourselves off from the world, it's about choosing how and with whom we want to live in it.

Knowing how to say no

In an age marked by hyper-connection, constant social pressure and a focus on permanent availability, saying no has become a revolutionary act. Yet this simple two-letter word has immense power when used wisely: it's an act of protection, lucidity and personal refocusing. In a minimalist approach to relationships, knowing how to say no is not only useful, it's vital. Because every yes you say involves a share of your energy, your time and your attention. And these resources are limited. Minimalism in relationships invites you to recognise that your energy is precious, and that it deserves to be invested in relationships that really nourish you, not in those that drain you.

Saying no doesn't mean rejecting the other person: it means choosing yourself

One of the reasons why so many people find it hard to say no is that they confuse refusal with a personal attack on the other person. They fear disappointing, hurting, being perceived as selfish or cold. But this fear stems from a misperception of limits. Saying no doesn't mean that you don't love someone, or that you never want to help them. It simply means: I'm listening to myself, I respect myself, and I'm making a conscious choice about what I'm able or willing to give at this precise moment. Learning to say no means coming back to yourself, to your own needs, to your own balance. It means recognising that you can't be a constant resource for others without emptying yourself.

A concrete example: a friend regularly asks you to talk about his problems, but never listens to you in return. If you always say yes, you become an emotional reservoir for him, but you betray yourself, because your need to be listened to and reciprocated is not honoured. Saying no in this context puts you back at the centre of the relationship. It's a clear signal: "I'm willing to help you, but not by sacrificing my own mental health." It's not coldness: it's personal ecology.

Relationship minimalism requires voluntary selection

In the minimalist logic, we purge what is superfluous, what clutters, what suffocates - and this also applies to relationships. Knowing how to say no becomes a sorting tool here. Not all relationships are created equal. Some make you grow, elevate you, inspire you. Others drag you down, make you anxious, make you feel guilty or leave you emotionally drained. Relationship minimalism encourages you to observe your interactions with lucidity, and to sort them out: which relationships nourish me? Which ones consume me?

But be careful: this sorting out is not brutal. It's not a matter of coldly cutting ties with everyone, but of adjusting your level of commitment, of saying no to certain dynamics, certain patterns or certain frequencies. Perhaps you won't cut all ties with a toxic person in your family, but you will decide to reduce your interactions, to stop exposing yourself to their repeated criticism. This more subtle type of no is often the most liberating

It's a no that restores your mental space, without necessarily breaking ties.

The art of saying no without feeling guilty

Learning to say no also means deconstructing the guilt that is deeply rooted within us. Since childhood, we've been taught that refusing is rude, that to be appreciated you have to be kind, helpful and always available. This conditioning pushes us to constantly over-adapt, to say yes even when our whole body is screaming no. The result? Chronic fatigue, silent frustration, a feeling of emptiness, even resentment. From this point of view, saying no means repairing an internal fracture. It means reclaiming your right to integrity. And that requires a gradual apprenticeship.

It is possible to say no gently, firmly and respectfully. There's no need to over-justify or feel obliged to explain everything. Here are some simple but powerful formulations:

- "Thank you for your offer, but I'm going to decline".
- "It's not possible for me this time".
- "I'd rather concentrate on something else at the moment.
- "I appreciate you thinking of me, but I'm going to say no.

The most important thing is not what you say, but the state of mind in which you say it. If your no comes from a place of inner clarity and self-respect, it will be received more easily. And even if the other person reacts badly, it's not your role to bear that reaction.

to bear that reaction. Your responsibility is to preserve your breathing space.

Saying no creates a virtuous circle

The more you learn to say no, the more you realise how much it clarifies your relationships. People who really love you understand your approach. They respect your limits. And above all, they reciprocate. By saying no to things that don't suit you, you create a healthier relationship model, based on authenticity rather than convenience or fear of conflict. You become more available for what really matters.

This virtuous circle also works within you: every no that you say correctly makes you stronger, more coherent and freer. You begin to live life on your own terms, building a social life that is chosen rather than imposed. Your yeses become more valuable, because they become sincere, meaningful commitments.

Knowing how to say no, as part of a minimalist approach to relationships, means reconciling self-love with the quality of relationships. It's not about rejecting the other person: it's about choosing yourself. It's not hurting: it's protecting. It's a silent but powerful affirmation: "I choose what I allow in my life". By learning to say no, you make room for what matters, eliminate what depletes, and create a human environment that is calmer, clearer and more aligned with who you are becoming.

Refocus on authentic connections

In a world where human interaction is multiplying on the surface but impoverishing at the core, it's becoming vital to sort out your relationships in order to preserve your energy, time and emotional integrity. Relational minimalism suggests that we reconsider the way we weave our social links: it's not about living in isolation, but choosing consciously with whom we build, who inspires us, who lifts us up. Refocusing on authentic connections means refusing to waste energy on lukewarm or unbalanced relationships, instead investing in those that have real meaning. It's a process of clarity, emotional sobriety and alignment.

1. Sorting your relationships like you sort your things

Just as material minimalism invites us to get rid of the superfluous and keep only the essential, relational minimalism encourages us to observe, without guilt, our relationships in terms of their quality, sincerity and reciprocity. This step requires us to be emotionally clear-headed: some relationships, even long-standing ones, may be toxic, unbalanced or simply obsolete. It's no mistake that certain people no longer have a place in our lives. We evolve, and so do our relationship needs.

They may be friendships maintained purely out of habit, family ties based on the fear of disappointing, or opportunistic acquaintances who draw on our resources without ever nourishing our being in return. Sorting out our relationships does not mean 'throwing out' others, but rather recognising the dynamics that are no longer beneficial. This allows us to reclaim our emotional space, like reorganising a cluttered room so that we can finally breathe.

2. Choose depth over dispersion

Modern culture often values the quantity of contacts: more friends on the networks, more messages exchanged, more social activities. Yet this hyper-connection is often an illusion. You can know a hundred people without really understanding any of them, or be surrounded by people without ever feeling seen. Refocusing on authentic connections means making a radical choice: choosing depth over dispersion.

It means focusing your energy on a few key relationships, where you can really express yourself without a filter, be vulnerable without fear, share without strategy. A single person with whom you feel fully understood is worth infinitely more than a whole network of fuzzy acquaintances. It takes courage, because making a deep commitment means exposing yourself, really listening, working through conflicts with maturity, and building over time. But that's where authenticity is born, in the solid bonds that become the pillars of our lives.

3. Learning to recognise genuine reciprocity

An authentic relationship is based on a balanced exchange of presence, listening and support. Relationship minimalism encourages us to observe whether our interactions are nourished in both directions or whether they function in a one-way fashion. Do you offer your attention to someone who never gives it back? Do you always make the first move, the only effort, the only concession? If so, perhaps it's time to readjust your boundaries.

It's not a question of keeping score, but of sensing whether the relationship dynamic is based on genuine mutual intent. Sometimes we insist on maintaining a relationship simply because we've known it for a long time, out of loyalty or fear of hurting someone's feelings. However, if this relationship is no longer based on sincere reciprocity, it becomes a burden. To distance oneself from it is to respect oneself and leave room for other, fairer connections to emerge.

4. Saying no to empty or destructive ties

In our need to belong, we sometimes agree to maintain ties that go against our equilibrium. This can take the form of being in groups where we feel invisible, forced social interactions where we have to play a role, or relationships where we are regularly belittled, manipulated or neglected. Relational minimalism teaches us that it's better to be alone than badly accompanied. It's a difficult truth to accept, but a profoundly liberating one.

To say no to an empty or harmful relationship is to affirm that your inner peace is non-negotiable. This "no" can be expressed by distancing yourself, withdrawing discreetly, or having an honest discussion. It is not a rejection of the other person, but a conscious choice to protect yourself. This stage requires discernment, self-honesty and often grief. But it opens up a precious path towards greater alignment, authenticity and peace.

5. Creating habits of deep connection with the right circles

Once you've sorted yourself out, another important step is to actively nurture the precious relationships you've chosen to keep. This doesn't mean always being available or stiflingly involved, but establishing simple, regular rituals that anchor the relationship in time and quality. This can take the form of a monthly dinner, a weekly phone call, a shared moment of silence, or even a simple, sincere message sent with care.

In these rituals, the quality of the moment shared is more important than its duration or frequency. It's not about ticking a box, but about being truly present. True presence is rare these days: it requires you to put down the phone, stop thinking about yourself, and open up fully to the other person. These micro moments of shared truth become bubbles of authenticity in the tumult of everyday life, anchors that remind us of what is truly essential.

6. Being authentic with yourself in order to be authentic with others

It's impossible to create an authentic connection with others if you don't first cultivate an honest relationship with yourself. Minimalism in relationships therefore begins with inner work: learning to listen to yourself, recognising your deep relational needs (need for support, sharing, freedom), identifying your emotional limits, understanding your wounds and defensive mechanisms.

The more you are internally aligned, the more naturally you will attract people who are compatible with your energy. The less you play a role, the more space you create for real connections. It's not about being perfect or invulnerable, but about becoming transparent with yourself: "this is how I feel", "this is what I'm looking for in a relationship", "this is what I don't want any more". This personal clarity is the foundation of any lasting connection.

7. Choosing solitude as a path to quality

Finally, refocusing on authentic connections also means making peace with solitude. Not as a sudden absence, but as a fertile space where we can find ourselves, repair ourselves and refocus. Relational minimalism sees solitude not as a punishment, but as an opportunity to rebuild. In silence, you hear your own voice again. And it's often in these moments of solitary alignment that the right relationships emerge, because we're no longer trying to fill a void, but to share a fullness.

Returning to authentic connections is a form of gentle rebellion against superficiality. It means taking care of yourself by taking care of your relationships. It means moving from quantity to quality, from the need to be surrounded to the joy of being understood, from social obligation to the freedom to love consciously. It's an art, a choice, a discipline, and above all an inner transformation that enables us to live more simply, more sincerely and more deeply.

Chapter 8: A minimalist wardrobe

The capsule wardrobe method

The accumulation of clothes is one of the most visible forms of over-consumption in our daily lives. In many homes, wardrobes are overflowing, hangers are bending under the weight of unused shirts, and yet the phrase "I've got nothing to wear" keeps cropping up. The solution to this paradox, which combines overabundance and dissatisfaction, lies in a method that's as simple as it is effective: Capsule Wardrobe. More than a clothing trend, it's a paradigm shift that aims to restore clothing to its rightful place as a tool for comfort, personal expression and mental freedom.

Origin and philosophy of the wardrobe capsule

The capsule wardrobe concept has its roots in the 1970s, introduced by Susie Faux, a London designer who proposed a wardrobe made up of a few essential, well-cut, high-quality pieces that were interchangeable and timeless. It wasn't until several decades later that

American blogger Caroline Joy, with her "Unfancy" project, brought the capsule back into fashion by popularising its practical application: living with around 33 items of clothing per season, including accessories and shoes.

But the capsule wardrobe is more than just a number or a predefined list. It's based on profoundly minimalist principles: reducing noise, simplifying choice, investing in what really matters, and eliminating the superfluous. It's a practice that questions our relationship with fashion, our image, consumerism and the freedom to be ourselves.

Why does adopting a minimalist wardrobe change your daily life? One

decision = less mental burden

Every item of clothing you lose is one less decision you have to make every morning. By limiting your options, you simplify your routine. This saving of time and mental energy is not insignificant: "decision fatigue" is a real psychological phenomenon, and it affects our mood, our efficiency and our well-being. A wardrobe capsule acts like an anti-chaos filter, allowing you to concentrate on what's essential: your day, your projects, your life.

Significant savings and rational consumption

Adopting a capsule wardrobe means breaking with the logic of impulse consumption. You no longer give in to purchases dictated by sales, social networks or boredom. Instead, we become active participants in our own consumption: each piece is chosen with intention, with sustainability in mind. This change translates into concrete savings in the short, medium and long term. What's more, it encourages an ethical approach: favouring responsible brands, avoiding fast fashion, and refusing to fuel the exploitation of the planet's human and ecological resources.

A refined, assertive personal style

The wardrobe capsule encourages you to explore who you really are, independent of fashion dictates. By narrowing down your options, you refine your style. You identify the cuts that make you stand out, the colours that illuminate your complexion and the fabrics in which you feel comfortable. This work of aligning your inner self (your tastes, your identity) with your outer self (your clothes) is a powerful act of reconnecting with yourself. You dress with intention, not automatism.

Concrete steps for creating your capsule wardrobe Step 1: The

great textile introspection

Before you even start sorting your clothes, take a moment to reflect on your relationship with clothing:

- Do you often buy out of boredom? Out of a need for novelty? Insecurity? ?
- What does your wardrobe say about your emotions?
- What clothes do you really wear? Which ones remain in the shadows?

These questions open the door to an emotional and practical sorting process that goes much deeper than simply tidying up. It's not just a question of throwing things away, but of freeing yourself from what's cluttering up your life physically and mentally.

Step 2: Take it all out, see it all, sort it all out

This can be a trying stage. Take out absolutely all your clothes, including shoes, accessories, bags and coats. Put them all together on a bed or in a large open space.

Then create four categories:

1. I love it, I wear it often, it's me: keep them without hesitation.
2. I love them, but I never wear them: question their place. Maybe it's time to part with them.
3. It doesn't fit any more, it's damaged or forgotten: give it away, sell it or recycle it.
4. I'm not sure: put these items in a "quarantined" box or bag and store them out of sight for 30 days. If you don't feel any loss, they're good to go.

This sorting is an act of liberation. It allows you to keep only what makes sense to you, and to create physical and mental space.

Step 3: Define your style, colours and needs

A successful capsule is based on consistency. Ask yourself:

- What are my favourite colours?
- What are my favourite cuts (high-waisted, loose, fitted)?
- What clothes give me confidence?
- Do I have a bohemian, classic, urban, sporty or minimalist style?

Then define a colour palette:

- 2 or 3 basic neutrals: black, white, grey, beige, navy blue, etc.
- 2 or 3 accent colours: khaki, rust, burgundy, mustard, etc.

This palette makes it easier to find harmonious combinations and avoid buying mistakes.

Also analyse your real needs:

- Office work? Is professional clothing compulsory?
- Regular or infrequent outings?
- Active or rather quiet lifestyle?

These are the elements that will guide your capsule.

Step 4: Compose your capsule by season

Here's a typical example for a capsule wardrobe for one season (spring or autumn):

Type of piece	Recommended number	Remarks
Tops (t-shirts blouses, fine jumpers)	7 à 9	Multiply the layers
Bottoms (jeans, skirts trousers)	4 à 6	Vary according to your needs
Dresses or overalls	2 à 3	For occasions or simplicity
Coats or jackets	2 à 3	A warm coat, a light jacket
Shoes	2 à 4	One pair for walking, one pair of dress shoes
Accessories (scarves, bags, belts)	3 à 5	Keep it simple and practical

Adapt this model to your lifestyle. The aim is for each piece to have a clear function and to be able to be combined with at least three other garments.

Step 5: Buy with intention, or not at all Once

you've put together your capsule, you can :

- Top it off with one or two pieces that are missing (e.g. a good pair of jeans or a neutral blazer).
- Decide not to buy anything and live the experience with what you have.
  you have.

If you buy:

- Buy one piece at a time.
- Always ask yourself: Does it go with everything else? Will I wear it at least 30 times?
- Choose natural materials, timeless cuts and ethical brands if possible.

The wardrobe capsule as a tool for inner transformation

Creating a wardrobe capsule is a profoundly transformative act. It's a return to oneself. You learn to get to know yourself better, to dress better, to lighten up from the gaze of others, to assert a simple, strong and calm identity. This process teaches us that freedom lies not in unlimited choice, but in the quality of our choices.

In our fast-paced lives, the capsule wardrobe offers us a space for slowness, reflection and coherence. It is a tool of applied minimalism that is both visible and symbolic. It reminds us that less is more, and that in the silence of the superfluous is born the essential.

Choose versatile, durable pieces

In a minimalist wardrobe, each item of clothing must be chosen with care, not on a whim or an impulse, but according t o its real purpose, its quality, its ability to be easily combined, and its longevity over time. Minimalist clothing is based on a philosophy of functionality, sobriety and durability, where quantity is replaced by relevance. The aim is to have fewer pieces, but more possibilities. To achieve this, two fundamental principles guide our clothing choices: versatility and durability.

1. Versatility: the cornerstone of an effective wardrobe

Versatility is the ability of a garment to adapt to different contexts, to be transformed by different combinations, and to meet several needs without having to make multiple purchases. In a minimalist logic, it is no longer a question o f owning a garment for each specific occasion (meeting, evening, weekend, holiday...), but rather of owning pieces capable of navigating between these universes with fluidity.

Take the example of a structured blazer in a neutral colour (black, beige, grey or navy blue). It can be paired with trousers for a professional outfit, slipped over a T-shirt and jeans for a casual outing, or worn over a light dress for a dinner party. So the same garment has three radically different uses, simply by changing the context and the accessories.

Similarly, a pair of raw, straight-cut jeans is a versatile essential: it lasts through the seasons, suits most body shapes and can be styled endlessly. With trainers and a sweatshirt, they're urban and casual; with loafers and a shirt, they're dressy without being strict. This type of piece is not dependent on trends, and fits naturally into a logic of stylistic efficiency.

In a minimalist wardrobe, each item of clothing should be paired with at least three to five other existing pieces. This principle, sometimes called the "3-pair rule", helps to avoid "orphan" clothes: those that you love but never wear because they don't go with anything. By following this rule, you create a coherent clothing system, where each element reinforces the versatility of the others.

2. Durability: a conscious long-term investment

Opting for sustainable clothing means choosing a healthy and responsible approach to consumption. It means prioritising quality over quantity, and seeing the purchase not as a fleeting pleasure, but as a useful and considered investment. Unlike the disposable clothes of fast fashion, durable garments are more resistant to washing and retain their shape, colour and appearance over time.

You can recognise sustainable clothes by several signs: they are often made from good quality natural or technical materials (wool, organic cotton, linen, Tencel, raw denim, etc.), with reinforced seams, solid finishes and a timeless cut. They don't follow passing fashions, but are rooted in a classic, timeless aesthetic that lasts through the years without seeming old-fashioned.

Investing in a good coat, sturdy jeans or a well-designed pair of leather shoes may cost more up front, but it will save you money in the long term. A €250 coat worn every winter for ten years costs €25 a year. On the other hand, a €60 coat that wears out in one winter has to be bought again regularly, which adds to the cost and the ecological footprint. Durability rhymes with profitability.

Minimalism also invites us to look beyond the label, to take an interest in the origin of the clothes, the working conditions of the workers, the impact of dyes or transport on the environment. Choosing a sustainable item often means supporting more ethical and humane fashion, where every purchase is a declaration of values.

3. Combining personal style, ethics and practicality

Choosing versatile, sustainable pieces doesn't mean giving up on your style or personality. On the contrary, it allows you to define your clothing identity more clearly. Minimalism helps you to get to know yourself better: what colours make me stand out? What clothes do I feel good in? What suits me on a daily basis?

By answering these questions, you build a wardrobe that is not standardised, but aligned with your needs and deepest tastes. This makes it possible to resist the effects of fashion, to stop indulging in compulsive buying and to free yourself from the pressure of always having to "have something new". A durable, versatile wardrobe becomes a tool for freedom: you know what you own, you save time every morning, and you make more space in your life and in your head.

4. Fewer objects, more presence

Finally, owning fewer clothes but choosing them more carefully reduces the mental burden of making choices. How many people feel paralysed when faced with a full wardrobe, unable to decide what to wear? An uncluttered, well-thought-out wardrobe, made up of compatible and reliable pieces, puts an end to this daily stress. It simplifies routines, frees up time and offers a feeling of clarity and lightness.

By only having clothes that you love, that you wear often, and that stand the test of time, you develop a healthier relationship with fashion. We detach ourselves from social pressure, cultivate gratitude for what we already have, and relearn to consume consciously. This discipline is reflected in other areas of life: money management, concentration, mental clarity and emotional balance.

Rethink your style in line with your values

In a minimalist approach, the wardrobe is no longer seen as a simple assembly of clothes, but as a reflection of our inner world, our identity and our deepest commitments. Rethinking your style in line with your values means asking yourself a fundamental question: "Does what I wear embody who I am and what I believe? Through this reflection, clothing becomes a tool for personal coherence, a tangible extension of our life ethic.

1. From unconscious consumption to aligned self-expression

For a long time, the way we dress has been dictated by external influences: fashion trends, social codes, the way others look at us, seductive shop windows and 'must-have' sales. This leads us to mindlessly accumulate clothes that often don't fit our bodies, our real style or our needs. The result: a wardrobe full to bursting, but a persistent feeling of "having nothing to wear".

Rethinking your style means breaking out of this cycle and adopting an introspective, conscious approach.
introspective and conscious approach. This means stopping for a moment to observe,

without judgement, what we actually wear on a daily basis. What clothes make us feel comfortable, confident and real? Which are systematically avoided?

? From this observation, we can gradually build a personal style that no longer seeks to follow fashion trends, but to express our authenticity. In this way, we move from a copy-and-paste style to an embodied style that speaks about us without saying a word.

2. Make your clothes an extension of your convictions

Minimalism invites us to align our possessions with our values. This principle fully applies to our clothes. For many people, this means taking an ethical and ecological turn. The fashion industry is one of the most polluting in the world, and much cheap clothing is produced in deplorable working conditions. Adopting a wardrobe that reflects your values often means choosing to stop contributing to this destructive system.

This can mean choosing sustainable, eco-friendly materials (such as linen, organic cotton or recycled wool), responsible brands, or buying second-hand. This change is not intended to make you feel guilty, but to liberate you. It gives meaning to each piece we choose. Wearing a garment becomes a gentle militant act, a small daily gesture that affirms: "I'm choosing a fairer, cleaner, more humane world". This approach gives our outfits an invisible but very real moral value, and reinforces our sense of inner coherence.

3. Simplify your wardrobe to gain mental and emotional freedom

Beyond ethical considerations, a minimalist wardrobe aligned with our values aims to reduce the number of pieces in favour of quality, versatility and relevance. It's not a question of imposing a fixed number of clothes on ourselves, but of aiming for a collection that corresponds to our real needs, our lifestyle and our climate.

our lifestyle and our climate. This voluntary reduction offers an often unsuspected benefit: mental and emotional relief.

Every morning, choosing what to wear becomes a simple, straightforward decision. Gone are the endless dilemmas, the outfits that no longer fit, the clothes we keep "just in case" but never wear. Everything we own is there because we chose it consciously, because it enhances us, and because it serves our daily lives. This simplification creates a feeling of order, control and serenity. We feel better about ourselves because we are in tune with ourselves, right down to the way we dress.

4. Building a personal style that lasts and evolves

A wardrobe aligned with our values is not frozen in time. It evolves with us, as we become more aware of ourselves, our experiences and our personal growth. Rethinking our style means accepting that clothing is a living part of our journey. Our tastes can change, our relationship with our body can evolve, and so can our daily lives. Minimalism teaches us to embrace this evolution without guilt or excess.

It also means taking the time to define our basic style. Do I prefer flowing or structured cuts? Neutral colours or natural tones? Loose-fitting or tight-fitting? What are the uniforms that suit me and in which I feel comfortable in all circumstances? From there, you can put together a capsule wardrobe, made up of key interchangeable pieces that are deeply personal to you. This personal style then becomes a silent signature, a way of presenting ourselves to the world with simplicity, clarity and pride.

5. Honouring each garment, extending its life, giving it meaning

Finally, rethinking your style in line with your values means learning to take care of your clothes, to give them attention and respect. In a world where it's easy to throw away what's damaged, the minimalist chooses to repair, sew and transform. They give their clothes a second life, cherish them and wear them with intention. Each item of clothing becomes a travelling companion, an object full of history and presence. This emotional bond, which we had lost through over-consumption, returns: we learn to love what we own again, because it looks like us and faithfully accompanies us.

Rethinking your clothing style with a minimalist approach is much more than a change of appearance. It's an act of reclaiming yourself, a way of living according to your deepest convictions. It means deciding not to dress to conform, but to respect yourself, to reveal yourself, and to contribute to a world more in line with your ideals. By integrating this coherence between style and values, each garment we choose becomes a tool of freedom, a silent messenger of our inner truth.

Part III - A Philosophy of Life

Chapter 9: Minimalism and personal development

Creating space for your passions

In a society where the pace is quickening, obligations are piling up and distractions are multiplying, it is becoming increasingly difficult to find the time, energy and clarity of mind needed to cultivate one's passions. Yet these activities that inspire us, awaken our enthusiasm and nourish our creativity are essential to our personal fulfilment. Minimalism, far beyond its material dimension, proposes a philosophy o f life that invites us to unclutter our daily lives to refocus our existence around what really matters. Creating space for our passions then becomes not only possible, but natural. It's an act of refocusing, o f reclaiming ourselves, a silent declaration: "I deserve time for what makes me come alive".

Clearing out material space: making room for what makes sense

The first step in creating space for your passions is often a concrete action: decluttering your physical environment. Our living, working and sleeping spaces are often saturated with objects we no longer use, which we keep out of habit, guilt or fear of lack. Each useless object represents an unconscious mental burden, a small source of distraction or annoyance. A cluttered desk, a cupboard full to bursting, a living room overrun with useless gadgets... all these things limit our ability to concentrate, to breathe, to feel free to express our creativity.

Minimalism invites us to sort things out honestly: what do I really need? What brings me joy? What objects actually support the activities that are important to me? This reflection often leads t o a revelation: a large proportion of our possessions are there for superficial or emotional reasons, but have no real use in our personal journey. By ridding ourselves of the unnecessary, we create a clearer, more functional environment, more conducive to the fulfilment of our passions.

Imagine a living space free of all superfluous objects, in which every object has a meaning, a function and a place. A minimal but cosy reading corner. A clean desk for writing, drawing and creating. A free cupboard, where you don't have to search for a notebook for twenty minutes.

a notebook or paintbrush for twenty minutes. This new physical space then becomes fertile ground for your creative activities and your heart's desire.

Reorganise your time: free up hours to reconnect with what drives you

Another form of decluttering, more subtle but just as essential, concerns our timetable. All too often, we feel overwhelmed, saturated, consumed by obligations, commitments, outside demands, incessant notifications... And yet, paradoxically, we all have the same amount of time: 24 hours a day. Time minimalism encourages us to become aware of how we use this precious time, and to redefine our priorities.

How much time do we spend on our phones each day, scrolling through content that leaves no trace? How many evenings are swallowed up by series watched mechanically for lack of energy or inspiration? How many reluctantly accepted tasks take us away from what we really enjoy doing? Creating space for our passions often requires a form of quiet courage: the courage to say no. No to the saturated agenda. No to the overloaded agenda. No to time-consuming distractions. No to unchosen social obligations.

It also means consciously scheduling time for yourself, just as you would schedule an important appointment. It could be half an hour a day to write. An hour a week to paint. One Saturday a month for a nature walk. These moments don't just happen: they need to be planned, protected and cherished. Minimalism teaches us that the quality of our lives does not depend on what we accumulate, but on how we live each moment. By learning to manage our time better, we can gradually transform our daily lives into a fertile space where our passions can be fully expressed.

Lightening the mental load: regaining inner clarity

Our minds are cluttered too. Repetitive thoughts, worries, comparisons, endless to-do lists, fear of not being up to the job... This inner turmoil forms a constant background noise that interferes with our ability to concentrate, feel and create. To allow our passions to emerge, we also need to make room in our minds.

Mental minimalism means simplifying our way of thinking: letting go of perfectionism, stopping trying to control everything, giving up constant multitasking. It means choosing depth over dispersion. It also involves practices such as meditation, conscious breathing, introspective writing and even regular periods of digital disconnection. These moments of self-assumed emptiness are not a waste of time: they are the cradle of our creativity. Because it's often in the silence, in the slowness, in the space left free, that the best ideas emerge, the right intuitions, the deep impulses towards a passion that we had forgotten.

By reducing inner noise, we rediscover our presence. And this presence is essential to nourish our passions, which require quality time, sincere attention and a deep connection to what we feel.

Reconnecting with what makes us tick

All too often, our passions are stifled by everyday life. We tell ourselves "I'll do it later", "when I've got the time", "when I'm less tired", "when I've got the right equipment". And the years go by. Minimalism reminds us that what makes us alive deserves a central place, not a secondary one. Our passions are not bonuses, extras or anecdotal hobbies: they are manifestations of our deepest essence. They are the activities in which time seems to stand still

They are the activities where time seems to stand still, where we feel fully ourselves, where we give the best of ourselves effortlessly.

Creating space for your passions is an act of self-love. It's about honouring that part of us that craves beauty, creation and discovery. It's sending a clear message to your spirit: "You are important. What you love has value. You have the right to fulfil yourself.

This sometimes means readjusting your whole life: changing your priorities, reorganising your home, reviewing your social relationships, rethinking your professional ambitions... but it's worth it. Because a life without passion is a life on automatic pilot. A life structured around your passions, however simple or modest, is a life that is lived, vibrant and deeply satisfying.

Getting back to basics: what really matters

In our society of over-consumption, hyper-connection and constant demands, we have gradually lost sight of what is really important. We are often overwhelmed by useless objects, parasitic thoughts, superficial relationships and obligations that don't resonate with our inner truth. Getting back to basics means starting a conscious process of refocusing on what truly nourishes our being: our values, our well-being, our authentic relationships and our life mission.

1. Distinguishing the necessary from the superfluous

Minimalism, as a philosophy of life, invites us to make a radical sorting out of all aspects of our existence.
in all aspects of our lives. It's not just a question of

It's not just about clearing the clutter from your physical space, but above all about clearing the clutter from your mind. This starts by asking ourselves a simple but powerful question: "What do I really need?" The answers vary from person to person, but they always reveal a profound truth: we need much less than what society pushes us to want. This return to the essentials frees us from the weight of accumulation, appearances and constant comparison.

2. Redefining our priorities

Getting back to basics means reconsidering our priorities with a clear head. In a minimalist logic, every choice becomes a statement of meaning. Personal development is rooted in conscious decisions: choosing time spent with loved ones over hours spent on social networks, preferring a rewarding activity to a passive distraction, or choosing a simple but aligned life over a prestigious but meaningless career. It's an invitation to move from a full life to a full life.

3. Living with intention

Minimalism is a school of intention. Every object, every relationship, every action must be examined through the prism of intention. Why do I keep this thing? Why do I associate with this person? Why do I pursue this activity? This regular questioning becomes a tool for personal transformation, because it encourages us to keep only what brings us joy, peace or growth. Living with intention means making the daily choice to nourish what really matters.

4. Quality rather than quantity

Our age glorifies 'always more': more possessions, more distractions, more visible success. But minimalism, combined with personal development, proposes a radically different approach: less is more. Fewer relationships, but deeper ones. Fewer activities, but more meaningful. Fewer objects, but better quality. This shift towards quality nurtures inner serenity and feeds a real sense of wealth, not material, but existential.

5. Reconnecting with the intangible essentials

By going back to basics, we rediscover that the most precious things can't be bought: silence, inner peace, time, love, nature, being present with oneself. These intangible elements, often relegated to second place, are nonetheless the source of lasting well-being. Minimalism opens the way to this rediscovery, by eliminating external noise to bring out what has always been there, deep within us.

6. An act of freedom and responsibility

Going back to basics is an act of courage. It means breaking with social injunctions, resisting the sirens of conformity, and daring to be simple in a world that scorns simplicity. But it's also an act of responsibility: towards yourself, because you're choosing a healthier, more conscious life; towards others, because you're putting an end to the logic of competition and appearances; towards the planet, because a minimalist life is naturally more ecological.

Going back to basics doesn't mean depriving yourself, it means freeing yourself. It means exchanging accumulation for clarity, agitation for peace, dispersion for coherence. By linking minimalism and personal development, we discover a philosophy of life that puts the human being, consciousness and simplicity back at the centre. Perhaps this return to the essential is, ultimately, a return to the self.

The link between minimalism and mindfulness

At first glance, minimalism and mindfulness seem to belong to different fields: one is concerned with the material environment, the other with inner experience. Yet they are intimately linked by the same quest: that of a more conscious, more balanced, more intentional life. One cannot exist without the other. Minimalism is the outward translation of a state of inner presence, while mindfulness is the foundation on which material deprivation can be approached with meaning and depth. Together, they form not just a method of living, but a veritable philosophy of existence.

1. Living intentionally: putting awareness back into every choice

The heart of minimalism lies not in having little, but i n choosing lucidly what you keep in your life. This choice presupposes a return to oneself. It's not a question of following a purified fashion, but of making an active, personal selection, in line with our deepest values. This sorting out is only possible when we are fully present to ourselves. This is where mindfulness plays an essential role.

Mindfulness involves paying deliberate attention to the present moment, without judgement. It invites us to observe our thoughts, emotions and impulses, and to become aware of the often automatic mechanisms that guide our daily lives. By developing this capacity for inner observation, we become better equipped to question our consumer behaviour:

– Why did I buy this object?
– Is it a real need or an emotional compensation?
– Do I keep it out of attachment or fear of lack?

Without awareness, we accumulate. With mindfulness, we choose. We move from reflex to intention, from filling to clarity. You take back control of your life, one choice at a time.

2. Decluttering as a path to inner peace

Living in a cluttered space, saturated with objects, notifications, noise and commitments, creates a dull mental fatigue. The brain is constantly in demand, scattered and uprooted from the present moment. Minimalism helps to reduce this background noise, not only in our physical environment, but also in our minds. External clutter is often a reflection of inner turmoil, and vice versa.

By freeing up our physical space, we open up a breach towards a deeper sense of calm. This apparent emptiness, far from being worrying, becomes a refuge for the soul. A space where we breathe better, think more clearly and feel more accurately. Mindfulness accompanies us on this journey: it teaches us to inhabit this emptiness with serenity, instead of compulsively filling it.

For example, taking the time to tidy a drawer, empty a cupboard or simplify your decor becomes a meditative act. This is no longer a utilitarian approach, but a practice of presence, a form of energetic purification. Each object that is eliminated becomes a calmed thought, each space freed up a new breath.

3. Reducing possessions to better hear your truth

Today's society pushes us to possess more and more, to be busier and busier, to respond to constant demands. In this never-ending stream, we end up losing sight of ourselves. Minimalism, nourished by mindfulness who am I really, apart from what I own, what I show, what I do?

When we let go of the superfluous, we begin to hear a subtler, more authentic inner voice. It's the whisper of our true aspirations, our deepest desires, our true being. But to hear this whisper, we need silence. Minimalism offers us this silence by reducing distractions. And mindfulness allows us to listen to this silence with attention, patience and kindness. Ask yourself regularly:

– Does this relationship uplift me?
– Does this activity really nourish my energy?
– Does this habit bring me closer to or further away from who I want to become?

These questions, asked with sincerity, are the seeds of lasting inner transformation. They put the power back in our hands. They allow us to redefine our priorities not in terms of the outside world, but in terms of our inner compass.

4. A slower pace for a fuller life

Minimalism and mindfulness both propose a radical paradigm shift: slowing down. In a world obsessed with speed, efficiency and profitability, choosing to slow down is an act of courage. It means taking the time to do things one at a time, to live them to the full, to savour every moment.

Drinking a coffee in silence, without a telephone. Listening to someone without thinking about their response. Walking without hurrying. Reading without interruption. Every gesture becomes a ritual of presence, a celebration of the moment. Quality takes precedence over quantity. We no longer chase time: we finally meet it.

This deliberate slowness makes for a denser, richer, more aligned life. It's an inhabited slowness, not a loss of productivity. Because in reality, the more we live with full awareness, the more effective we become at what's essential. The superfluous evaporates. What we keep, we live with intensity.

5. Minimalism and mindfulness: a synergy in the service of inner freedom

Ultimately, minimalism and mindfulness are not techniques to be applied on an ad hoc basis, but pillars of a new relationship with oneself, with others and with the world. They are powerful allies in personal development, because they free us from both visible chains (accumulation, distractions, obligations) and invisible chains (fears, conditioning, mental automatisms).

Live with less to be more. Possess less to feel more. Lighten up to love better, choose better, live better. That's the promise of this synergy. It guides us towards a form of inner wealth, far more precious than any external accumulation.

Chapter 10: Living intentionally

Setting clear priorities

One of the most powerful foundations of an intentional life is the ability to consciously define one's priorities. It's an act of lucidity and personal sovereignty. In a society where we are constantly bombarded with opportunities, solicitations, distractions and distractions,

distractions and external expectations, it's extremely easy to lose track of what's really important. Setting clear priorities means refusing to let the outside world decide for us how our time, energy, attention and life should be spent. It means stating forcefully: "This is what's important to me, and I'm going to build my life around it.

1. Defining your core values

Before even talking about concrete goals or choices, we need to get back to the essence of what drives us: our values. Clear priorities are not set in a vacuum. They are rooted in an intimate understanding of what we consider to be right, beautiful and essential. Yet very few people take the time to stop and pinpoint their true values. We're often content to go with the flow, to pursue 'important' things because we've been taught that they are: a prestigious career, a good salary, a well-ordered family life. But are these goals our own, or have society chosen them for us?

To answer t h i s question, we need to undertake some honest introspection. What makes me tick? What gives me a sense of fulfilment? What experiences have made me feel fully alive? By identifying what makes sense to us - freedom, authenticity, creativity, transmission, love, exploration, justice - we lay the foundations for our system of priorities. Because a priority only has value if it is aligned with what we deeply want to live and embody.

2. Making choices and accepting renunciations

Setting priorities is not simply a matter of drawing up a list of things we'd like to achieve. It's also, and above all, about making choices, which inevitably involves giving up certain things. And that's often where the problem lies. Because we live in a culture of the unlimited, of "anything is possible", of "you can have it all". This idea, seductive on the surface, is a dangerous illusion. In truth, every sincere 'yes' requires a thousand courageous 'no's'. Saying yes to a simple, aligned life means saying no to over-consumption, to social frenzy, to family or professional expectations that disconnect us from ourselves.

Setting clear priorities means sorting, simplifying and putting an end to dispersion. This may mean refusing certain invitations, delegating responsibilities, ending commitments that no longer resonate with our heart, or even leaving a toxic environment. We must dare to adopt this form of benevolent radicalism: one that protects our vital energy and honours our true aspirations. We can't do everything. But we can do deeply what is essential, and that's what gives meaning to our lives.

3. Translating our priorities into our agenda

Once the major priorities have been defined on the basis of our values and our deepest aspirations, the crucial moment comes when we have to translate them into everyday life. Because a priority that remains theoretical, mental or spiritual, without concrete translation into the timetable, is just wishful thinking. Living intentionally means that our days must reflect our inner commitments. If health is a priority, then exercise, rest and mindful eating should feature in the diary in the same way as an important business appointment. If writing, meditation or spending time with loved ones are priorities, they must have a fixed, stable, protected place in the week's schedule.

This often means completely rethinking the way you manage your time. We no longer set our priorities "when we have time", but reserve the best times for them, those when we are most concentrated, calmest and most available. This also means rethinking our relationship with digital distractions, social networks social networks, and urgent but unimportant tasks. We have to learn to distinguish between what's essential and what's just noisy, and to put our energy in the right place. An intentional life is one in which every minute has a direction, a meaning, a chosen destination.

4. Practise regular refocusing

Priorities are not set in stone. They evolve over time, with the seasons of life, personal circumstances, discoveries and inner transformations. What is a priority at 20 may not be at 35, and what seemed crucial yesterday may lose its relevance tomorrow. That's why it's essential to put in place a regular practice of refocusing. This can take the form of weekly, monthly or annual reviews, where we ask ourselves a few simple but powerful questions:

− Am I still aligned with what I'm doing?
− Do my daily actions really serve my priorities?
− Have I let distractions or habits take control of my time?
− What do I want to adjust, delegate or stop doing?

This return to oneself is an act of clarity and honesty. It allows us to correct our course before we stray too far, to realign our daily lives with our deepest intentions. It's a kind of regular inner dialogue between the pilot and the compass. It's not a question of constantly questioning everything, but of ensuring that the course remains correct, alive and nourishing.

5. Creating an energy hierarchy

Finally, it's essential to recognise that not all priorities are of equal intensity and energy. intensity and energy. Some things can be done every day, others once a week, others once a week.

others once a week, and still others once a year. So it's useful to prioritise according to frequency, impact and feasibility. This helps to avoid mental overload and the guilt of not 'doing everything'. Living intentionally does not mean living in "maximum productivity" mode, but living coherently, fluidly and consciously.

Creating this energetic hierarchy means recognising that some areas of our lives require a deep and abiding commitment (for example, taking care of our mental health or our children), while others can be nurtured by one-off but intentional actions (such as an annual trip, an art project, a spiritual retreat). By placing priorities in appropriate time cycles, we free up space, gain serenity and, above all, respect the natural rhythm of life.

Setting clear priorities means taking back the reins of your life with calm, determination and humility. It means moving from 'reactive' to 'creative' mode. It means making the conscious choice not to live on automatic pilot, but to live each day to the full in the certainty that what we do is in line with who we are. This requires discernment, courage and discipline, but the benefits are immense: greater clarity, less stress, a life richer in meaning and fulfilment. By cultivating this practice on a daily basis, we transform our existence into a work of art - a work that is chosen, thought out and loved.

Define your values and live them

Living intentionally isn't just about wanting more control over your life; it's a profound process that begins with a fundamental question
What's really important to me? Even before setting goals

or plan actions, it's essential to define what, in our eyes, gives value to existence. Without this, all decisions, no matter how rational or productive, run the risk of being disconnected from our true identity. This is where working on values comes into its own.

1. Understanding the nature of values: invisible but fundamental pillars

Values are neither passing fancies nor fashionable opinions. They are the invisible foundations on which we build our lives. They are non-negotiable principles that determine h o w we perceive the world, enter into relationships, react to events and make choices. Unlike objectives, which are specific, measurable and time-defined, values are cross-cutting: they are expressed in all areas of life - relationships, work, health, leisure, personal development.

For example, if a person places a high value on autonomy, this value will be expressed in their desire to have a flexible job, in their preference for balanced relationships and in their desire to manage their own finances. Value therefore acts as a slow interpreter of reality. It influences our priorities, our behaviour and even our emotions, often unconsciously. So misidentifying our values is like letting someone else write the script of our lives.

2. Why living without clear values leads to inner incoherence

Not knowing your own values is like steering a ship without a rudder: you move forward, you make efforts, you go with the flow, but you don't know where you're going or whether it makes sense for you. This leads to a life dominated by the outside world - parents' expectations, social norms, comparisons on social networks - instead of a life based on personal authenticity.

This lack of clarity is often at the root of many forms of malaise: chronic procrastination, inner conflicts, existential emptiness, burn-out, widespread anxiety. These symptoms are not inevitable: they are often signals of a life that is off-centre, i.e. a life in which the individual no longer feels aligned with themselves. A person who deeply values inner peace but engages in a stressful, confrontational or competitive job will experience a permanent tension between their external environment and their inner world. It is this dissonance between actions and values that wears you down, exhausts you and makes you lose the desire to live life to the full.

3. Identifying your true values: essential introspective work

You can't define your values by consulting a ready-made list or adopting the popular beliefs of the moment. It's an introspective, personal process, often demanding but fundamental. It involves distinguishing between the inherited values inculcated by family, culture and school and the chosen values, i.e. those that we have experienced, lived and confirmed through experience.

Here are some practical ways of doing this:

- Think back to moments of profound fulfilment: What were you doing? What emotions did you feel? What quality of yourself was at stake? Was it courage, freedom, connection, creativity?
- Analyse your anger and hurt: Every time you've felt deeply hurt or indignant, one of your values has probably been violated. For example, if you feel unjustified rage at a harmless lie, it may be that truth and integrity are essential pillars for you.
- Take stock of your lifelong desires: What kind of people do you admire? Why do you admire them? What causes move you? What activities

that totally absorb you and in which you feel 'at home'?

- Use contrast: Imagine the worst version of yourself. What behaviours, attitudes or contexts do you deeply dislike? Contrast often reveals the opposite: what you deeply aspire to.

At the end of this exploration, it's a good idea to identify between 5 and 7 cardinal values. Anything less and you risk being too rigid; anything more and you'll spread yourself too thin. These values form a stable identity foundation around which to build a fully aligned life.

4. Embodying your values: from theory to daily practice

Identifying your values is pointless if they don't come alive. All too often, people display their values like slogans ("I'm an authentic person", "I value the family") but live in contradiction to them. Living your values means embodying them in every decision, every relationship, every project. This requires vigilance, courage and consistency.

Let's take an example: a person who identifies the value of "health" as central but who smokes, neglects their diet and doesn't move their body is living in dissociation. This internal fracture can only lead to latent malaise and even a loss of self-esteem. Conversely, aligning our behaviour with our values creates internal coherence, a feeling of unity that boosts confidence and serenity.

Living your values on a daily basis means :

- Making aligned choices, even if this means short-term losses (eg.
  Making aligned choices, even if this means short-term losses (e.g. leaving a well-paid job that is at odds with your principles).

- Developing concrete habits that embody your values (e.g. if you value learning, devote time each week to reading, exploring and training).
- Say no clearly when a situation, proposal or relationship d o e s not meet your life standards.
- Adjust regularly: life evolves, and your values may be nuanced and prioritised differently depending on the season of your life. The important thing is to stay actively in touch with them.

5. The benefits of a life aligned with your values: a foundation of power
power

When we live in deep harmony with our values, a radical inner change takes place. It's not just a psychological comfort, i t 's an existential transformation. We no longer live on the surface of things, in reaction or flight, but in depth, in serene clarity. Decisions become more fluid, doubts less paralysing, goals more motivating. Why ? Because we know why we're acting. We have a direction. A meaning. A reason for being.

What's more, this consistency attracts respect, trust and truer relationships. You no longer need to play a role or please at all costs. You become integral: who you are, what you say and what you do converge.

Finally, living by your values prepares you better to face trials. Because even in the storms, you know what you stand for, what you stand for and what you refuse to betray. This foundation becomes an unshakeable inner strength, an anchor that enables you to get through setbacks, bereavements and break-ups without losing your way.

Living intentionally begins with an act of lucidity: taking the time to identify what is essential for you. It's not external circumstances that define the quality of our lives, but our ability to respond to them with integrity. Defining our values, and then living them with courage, gives us the opportunity to stop reacting to the world, and to meet it with full awareness. It means making our life not an accident or a series of routines, but a coherent whole, faithful to our heart and our deepest truth.

Less, but better: the key to an aligned life

A philosophy of the essential in a world of dispersion

We live in an age where abundance is glorified. The accumulation of goods, projects, relationships and information seems to have become an indicator of success. We congratulate those who lead several lives in one, who fill their days to the point of exhaustion, who leave no gaps in their schedules. Yet this quest for 'always more' leaves behind a trail of mental fatigue, inner confusion and, often, a profound sense of emptiness. Living intentionally means making precisely the opposite choice: it means opting for clarity rather than overload, direction rather than dispersion, depth rather than superficiality.

Saturation distances us from ourselves

The more we fill our material, emotional and mental space, the harder it becomes to hear our own inner voice. It's as if every useless object, every unchosen obligation, every digital distraction becomes a silent parasite that jams our inner frequency. And this interference has

We no longer know what we really want. We act by reflex, we consume to escape, we run without knowing where we're going. By choosing to live with fewer objects, fewer activities and fewer demands on our time, we're not just 'emptying out': we're creating a sacred space, a fertile silence in which what really is us can finally emerge.

Intention as a selection filter

"Less is more" is based on a logic of conscious selection. This means that every element of our lives is filtered through a simple but powerful grid
Does it serve my well-being? Does it nurture my values? Does it correspond to who I want to be? When applied without concession, this filter acts as a revealer. It brings to light what is authentic in our lives, and what is there out of habit, conformity or fear of lack. Little by little, we learn to say no: no to activities that no longer nourish us, no to energy-guzzling relationships, no to possessions that weigh us down. But above all, every no becomes a yes to ourselves.

From quantity to quality: a radical transformation

Moving from a life based on quantity to one focused on quality is no small adjustment. It's a radical transformation in the way we think, choose and live. It takes courage, because this choice forces us to slow down, to give up external validation, to stop 'proving' by performance or agitation that we exist. But this transformation opens the door to a deeper joy: the joy of doing few things, but doing them with intensity, with love, with presence. It's no longer productivity that defines us, but the relevance and alignment of our actions. A simple walk becomes a moment o f communion with ourselves. A task well done becomes an act of offering. A sincere word becomes an act of presence.

An aligned life is an intentional life

Living intentionally means refusing to suffer. It means once again becoming the author of your daily life, the architect of your space, the curator of your priorities. This way of life leaves nothing to chance: it requires you to examine every aspect of your existence with a clear head. How do I spend my time? Where does my money go? Who do I spend my evenings with? What kind of content do I consume? How much energy do I put into my projects? As we sharpen this awareness, life ceases to be a series of random events: it becomes a work in progress. And it's precisely by reducing the superfluous that we begin to see the clear lines of the masterpiece we carry within us.

Less is more: the power of refocusing

The magnificent paradox of this approach is that by doing less, you become more. More present. More aligned. More alive. By reducing external noise, we increase our inner resonance. You stop living on the surface of yourself and go down to the core of your being. This process requires patience, because it's not a sudden change, but a succession of small adjustments, of gentle renunciations, of gradual sorting out. You lighten your living space, then your schedule, then your mind. And one day, almost without realising it, you feel light, centred, aligned, as if every element of your life were clicking into place.

Resistance to emptiness: an obstacle to overcome

It's natural to feel a form of resistance when it comes to sorting things out, slowing down or giving up. Emptiness is frightening. It evokes boredom, solitude and lack. That's why so many people prefer to stay in an uncomfortable state of overflow rather than risk calm. Yet this emptiness is actually a sacred space: it's the hollow necessary for all creation, for all rebirth. It is the equivalent of the blank page for the writer, of the ploughed earth for the gardener. It's in the emptiness that clear ideas, deep inspirations and sincere desires are born. Learning to love this emptiness, to move through it with confidence, is a major emotional skill in an intentional life.

Alignment as a source of inner peace

When we live "less but better", we live in alignment. This means that our outward actions correspond to our inner truth. There's no more double talk, no more silent compromise, no more masks to wear. This coherence, this unity between who we are, what we think and what we do, is the source of profound peace. A peace that doesn't depend on external circumstances, because it's rooted in fidelity to oneself. We no longer need to go fast, to do everything, to have everything. You just have to be there, fully, in the moment, in what you've chosen, in what you love.

Adopting the philosophy of "less but better" means making a daily commitment to yourself. It's not a goal to be achieved once and for all, but a journey. Every day, we are tempted to fall back into automatism, into dispersion, into "too much". And every day we have the opportunity to go back to basics, to refocus our energy, to choose again what really matters. It is this repetition, this daily return to ourselves, that transforms an intention into a way of life and an ordinary life into a work that is aligned, joyful and free.

Chapter 11: Minimalism and spirituality

Emptiness as openness

In the world of Minimalism, the void is not simply the absence of objects or noise, but a subtle presence, an energy in itself. It embodies a form of mental, emotional and physical space that has not been invaded or conquered, and which in fact allows something deeper to emerge. It's a deliberate retreat from the superfluous to make room for the essential. In this sense, emptiness is not a loss, but a creative power. It is fertile silence, inner calm, sacred space. This emptiness may at first seem frightening, especially to a mind conditioned to fill every moment, every corner, every silence. Yet it is in this emptiness that minimalism and spirituality meet: both invite us to stop occupying and start truly inhabiting.

Philosophically and spiritually, emptiness is a gateway to the deeper self. In Taoism, the concept of "Wu Wei" - action through non-action - is based on the ability not to force things, to leave empty space so that things can follow their natural course. Emptiness is seen as the condition for all inner transformation. It is not a question of filling up, but of disidentifying oneself from accumulation and agitation. In Buddhism, emptiness (or shunyata) does not mean nothingness, but the absence of fixation, **the** absence of a solid ego, **the** fluidity of existence. This emptiness is the very openness to compassion, wisdom and awakening. The spiritual minimalist adopts this vision: he learns to live in relationship with emptiness, not to lose himself in it, but to find himself in it.

On a more practical, day-to-day level, cultivating emptiness means choosing not to overload ourselves with objects, commitments or digital or emotional stimuli. For example, purifying your interior means creating an environment that breathes, that lets energy, light and attention circulate. It's not just a visual coquetry, it's a discipline of space that reflects an inner clarity. Less furniture means more movement. Fewer distractions mean more silence to listen to. Fewer objects mean more presence in every gesture. This emptiness, although discreet, becomes active, almost alive: it becomes the container of our consciousness, the fertile ground of our attention.

But this relationship with emptiness requires courage. Because emptiness confronts. It brings to light what we hide behind clutter: our fears, our wounds, our need to be reassured by the outside world. In this sense, emptying a room, unsubscribing from a network, saying no to a useless invitation, is not a simple logistical action. It's an act of inner resistance against dispersion. It's an invitation to be alone with ourselves, without mask, without décor, without pretense. And therein lies the transformation: emptiness becomes the school of presence. It teaches us to be in the moment, to breathe space, not to run away from what we feel. Paradoxically, it becomes the densest and truest fullness.

This emptiness is not passive. It is creative. It leaves room for the emergence of new perceptions, new awarenesses and more authentic visions of life. It reconnects you with your intuition, with your breath, with what we sometimes call "inner guidance". Where agitation and overflow drown out the truth, emptiness illuminates it. It allows us to hear the tiniest things: the right idea, a deep need, an obvious fact that emerges silently. It is in silence that wisdom speaks. In emptiness, we rediscover the ability to listen, not only to others, but above all to ourselves and to the living world around us.

Finally, living with emptiness as an opening means embracing a life that is less controlled, but more aligned. It means trusting the undefined space, the unplanned, the naturally emerging. It's about cultivating the art of letting go and being available. This way of life may seem uncomfortable to the ego, because it's based on uncertainty and lack of control. But for the soul, it offers a deep breath. A freedom to be, at last, in all its simplicity. A quiet joy that depends on nothing.

Detachment and inner peace

1. Detachment: inner liberation, not renunciation

In the context of spiritual minimalism, detachment should not be understood as an escape from reality or emotional indifference. On the contrary, it is a deeply conscious process that aims to regain power over what we give our attention, energy and inner peace to. Too often, we think we are defined by what we own, by our relationships, by our social image, or even by our ambitions. This kind of attachment builds a conditional, fragile self, dependent on constantly changing external circumstances. From this point of view, detachment is a radical act of inner sovereignty: it means refusing to let our happiness depend on what is beyond our control.

This does not mean renouncing all relationships or living without possessions. Rather, it means transforming our relationship with things and people. For example, instead of buying compulsively to fill a void, we choose each object for its real functional or aesthetic value, and not for what it symbolically promises (status, power, recognition). In our relationships, we learn to love without excessive attachment, i.e. without wanting to possess the other person or make them bear the burden of our emotional security. This detachment opens up an inner space from which a new, freer, lighter and more authentic way of living can emerge.

The spiritual dimension of minimalism encourages us to sort out not only our wardrobes, but above all our mental dependencies. Attachment is not just material: it can take the form of a constant need for validation, an attachment to one's image, to one's past, or to limiting thought patterns. Learning to detach yourself from them also means learning to defuse your ego, to stop defining yourself solely by what you do, what you own or what you show. This process doesn't happen overnight, but it is profoundly liberating, because it gives space back to the 'true self', the one that exists beyond social roles or possessions.

2. Inner peace: the reward of conscious self-denial

When we embark on the path of detachment, a subtle but powerful transformation takes place: the gradual emergence of lasting inner peace. Unlike the temporary peace brought on by external pleasure or success, this peace is not dependent on anything external. It comes from a stable state of presence, a refocusing on what's essential and an alignment with what makes sense to us. It's a peace that needs no justification. It manifests itself in the silence of the mind, in the acceptance of the present as it is, in the absence of struggle against ourselves.

This peace is made possible by stripping things away. By eliminating sources of distraction, overload or constant comparison, we find an inner space of clarity. This emptiness, initially feared and often associated with boredom or loss, turns out to be fullness: fullness of self, fullness of awareness, fullness of calm. Where the restlessness of the outside world fails to fill us, this peace becomes a solid refuge. It allows us to welcome our emotions without drowning in them, to experience the unexpected without becoming unbalanced, and to listen to others without losing ourselves in their projections.

Inner peace is not a fixed or unrealistic state. It coexists with challenges, responsibilities and sometimes even pain. But it allows us to face them differently. When the mind is no longer torn by a thousand parasitic thoughts, it becomes possible to respond rather than react. This difference is essential. Responding to life from a place of calm and clarity transforms every daily gesture into a conscious, almost sacred act. Minimalism then becomes a gateway to a lived spirituality, embodied in the simplicity of each moment.

3. Freedom through emotional autonomy

Detachment, when integrated into a minimalist and spiritual lifestyle, is the path to true emotional autonomy. This autonomy does n o t mean that we no longer feel anything or that we become insensitive, but that we are no longer slaves to our emotions or desires. We stop looking outside for what can only be found inside: recognition, security, unconditional love, wholeness. This requires a profound and often uncomfortable process of self-discovery, as it involves unlearning old mental habits, deconstructing beliefs and facing up to our own dark areas.

This inner freedom becomes a foundation. We no longer live in constant fear of losing what we have, or of not getting what we want. We no longer allow ourselves to be manipulated by commercial strategies that exploit our insecurities. We become the actors of our choices, in line with our deepest values. What was once seen as a sacrifice becomes a liberation: we discover the pure joy of being self-sufficient, of living a life in alignment, and of not needing anything to be well - not in a retreat, but in quiet power.

4. Contagious peace: radiating rather than convincing

When detachment is cultivated and inner peace takes root and lasts, we become an anchor for others. This peace doesn't need to be justified; it radiates naturally. You can feel it in the way you speak, look and act. It's not there to convince or impose a vision, but to inspire by silent example. In a world saturated with noise, social pressure, anger and agitation, a person who is internally calm becomes a landmark. Their calm becomes a balm for others, their sobriety a gentle provocation to re-evaluate their own excesses.

This radiance is not an objective in itself, but a natural consequence of the minimalist spiritual path. The more we detach ourselves from the ego, the more we become capable of serving without expectation, loving without condition, acting without pride. Inner peace becomes a powerful tool for collective evolution, because it shows that a different relationship to life is possible: slower, more conscious, more aligned. It's not a utopia, but a demanding path that is built step by step, in each choice, each conscious renunciation, each moment of silence that we agree to live fully.

Minimalism in the great spiritual traditions

Far from being a contemporary fad inspired by Scandinavian interior design or personal development trends, minimalism is an ancestral posture, rooted in humanity's greatest spiritual traditions. These traditions, whether Eastern or Western, monotheistic or philosophical, have always seen voluntary simplicity as a profound act of wisdom. Because external wealth is often a screen for inner wealth, and too many possessions, commitments or desires, an obstacle to peace of mind. In every major spiritual tradition, there is an appreciation of the value of simplicity, moderation and purity, not as a punishment but as a liberation. Minimalism is a path to the essential, a call to verticality, a way of removing what clutters to reveal what uplifts.

1. Buddhism: detachment as liberation from suffering

In Buddhism, minimalism takes a particularly explicit and structured form. The Buddha himself, Siddhartha Gautama, was a prince who abandoned his palace, wealth, pleasures and comforts in search of a deeper truth. This initial renunciation is the foundation of the entire Buddhist approach.
the understanding that suffering (dukkha) arises from attachment to ephemeral things - possessions, relationships, sensations. The path to enlightenment is therefore a gradual stripping away of these attachments.

In the Theravāda tradition, the Buddhist monk owns almost nothing. The Vinaya, the monastic code of conduct, deliberately limits possessions to a few essential items: three robes, an alms bowl, a razor, a needle and a water filter. This stripping down of possessions is not a punitive asceticism, but a means of removing the distractions of the world in order to devote oneself to the essentials: meditation, observation of the mind, understanding of non-self (anattā) and impermanence (anicca).

Spiritual minimalism in Buddhism is also internal: it involves simplifying the mind, reducing mental agitation and abandoning useless desires. Fewer possessions, fewer stimuli, fewer distractions for greater peace, greater clarity, greater inner freedom. Buddhism reminds us that true luxury is that of a peaceful consciousness, undisturbed by greed or fear of loss.

2. Christianity: voluntary poverty and inner wealth

In the Christian tradition, particularly in the Gospels, sobriety of life is a constant call. Jesus of Nazareth lived simply, walked among the humble, and preached self-emptying as a path to salvation: "It is harder for a rich man to enter the kingdom of God than for a camel to go through the eye of a needle". (Matthew 19:24). This verse sums up some radical wisdom: material abundance, far from being a blessing, can become a trap, because it weighs down the heart and turns people away from God.

The first Christians shared their possessions, lived in communities of solidarity and gave alms. But it was with the monastic movements, from the 3rd century onwards, that Christian minimalism became a total vocation. Figures such as Saint Anthony of the Desert and Saint Benedict left the world to live in prayer, poverty, silence and simple work. They took a vow of poverty not out of rejection of the material world, but out of a desire for profound communion with God, freed from the chains of possession.

Saint Francis of Assisi is the most emblematic example. The son of a wealthy merchant, he chose to beg, to live with the poor and to be in direct contact with nature. He advocated simple, unadorned joy, an existence that was bare but full of gratitude. From this perspective, minimalism becomes an act of love: by renouncing the superfluous, we make room for the essential, for others, for relationships, for transcendence.

3. Hinduism: Simplicity and the quest for the absolute

Hinduism, vast and complex, also proposes a profound appreciation of simple living and detachment. Vairagya, or detachment, is a central quality of wise Hindu. This detachment does not mean indifference, but mastery of desire: no longer being possessed by objects, emotions or relationships.

In the traditional order of the life (the ashramas), the ultimate stage the sannyasa consists of renouncing everything to devote oneself to the spiritual search. The sannyasin leaves his home, his family, his possessions and sometimes even his name. They live in nature, possessing only the essentials (often a simple garment, a stick and a bowl), and practise meditation, the study of sacred texts and contemplation of the divine.

This radical choice is seen as a liberation from illusion (maya). By abandoning the world of forms, the sage turns towards *Brahman*, the Absolute, beyond appearances. Hindu minimalism is therefore not an aesthetic, but an inner asceticism, a return to what is permanent, stable and true. It is a complete emptying of material, emotional and mental clutter to enable the realisation of Sō'ham: "I am That", the recognition of one's divine identity.

4. Sufism: Sobriety turned towards Love

In Sufism, the mystical current of Islam, minimalism takes on a loving hue. Sufis seek to purify their hearts so that they become mirrors in which the divine light is reflected. To do this, they must remove everything that stands in the way: pride, passions, attachments and, of course, material excess.

The notion of zuhd, which can be translated as "detachment" or "asceticism", consists of living soberly while keeping one's heart available to God. Sufis are not necessarily poor, but they act as if they owned nothing. They live in the world without being prisoners of it. They may be shopkeepers, craftsmen or married, but their hearts are not attached to passing things. Everything he owns is considered a sacred deposit, to be used with gratitude and generosity.

For many Sufis, true wealth is love: Ishq. A heart cluttered with material desires cannot contain this divine love. Minimalism thus becomes an act of purification, a self-effacement before the greatness of the Beloved. Mystical poets such as Rûmî or Al-Hallaj sang of this total renunciation, this extinction of the ego, to become one with the Presence.

5. Taoism: living in harmony with natural simplicity

Taoism, the age-old Chinese spiritual tradition, is based on the idea that nature itself is harmonious, fluid and balanced. By deviating from this, man creates his own suffering. To rediscover harmony, we need to return to original simplicity, to the spontaneity of life, to moderation. Lao Tzu's Tao Te King is a hymn to sobriety: "He who is content with little is truly rich".

Wu Wei, the central principle of Taoism, is often translated as "non-action", but it actually means "acting without effort", "acting in accordance with the natural flow of things". This implies a simple, uncluttered life, free from the superfluous. The Taoist sage does not seek to dominate the world, to accumulate or to shine. He prefers shadow to light, silence to noise, slowness to haste.

Taoist minimalism praises the natural, the spontaneous and the invisible. The less we possess, the more we feel. The less he imposes, the more he influences. In this vision, simplicity is not a rigid discipline, but a flexible, adaptive form of freedom. Living lightly means tuning into the rhythm of life and finding peace in the unforced.

All these traditions, despite their cultural and doctrinal differences, converge on a common truth: human beings find their greatness not in accumulation, but in stripping things away. Minimalism, in its spiritual essence spiritual essence, is not a deprivation, but a refocusing. It frees up space, internally and externally, so that the sacred can emerge.

To adopt this vision today, in a world saturated with consumerism and distraction, is to reconnect with an age-old wisdom. It means consciously choosing to live less full but more profound, less possessive but more present. It means turning every simple gesture into a sacred act, every emptiness into a call to presence, every renunciation into a return to the essential.

Conclusion

Throughout these pages, we have untangled the threads of our attachments, shed light on the shadows that clutter conceals, and given new meaning to simple, sometimes forgotten gestures. We have discovered that minimalism is neither a cold aesthetic nor an exercise in deprivation, but an art of living consciously, a philosophy that reconciles us with what is essential.

In a world saturated with stimuli, where every moment seems to be in demand, every space invaded, every silence filled, minimalism is an act of peaceful resistance. It is a bold choice: that of depth over surface, of quality over quantity, of slowness over haste. It's a gentle but firm cry against hyper-consumption, a lucid response to modern anxiety, a way of refocusing in a time of widespread noise.

Minimalism, as you've explored here, doesn't stop at the door of your house or the screen of your phone. It infuses all spheres of life: it transforms the way you think, dress, spend, love and choose. It teaches you to reclaim your time, your attention and your energy. It frees you from what you thought was necessary to help you discover what's really vital.

But this path is not linear. It's not about becoming perfect, or following rigid rules. It's about learning to live with intention, in each moment. It's about asking yourself not "do I have enough? but rather "does this serve me? does it make me happy? is it in line with my deepest values? This intimate, evolving process will guide you towards a lighter, infinitely richer life.

You'll discover that by having less, you don't lose anything: you gain space, calm, presence and clarity. You gain the ability to listen to what your heart has been whispering for so long, but which the din of the superfluous was stifling. You once again become the master of your story, free to write each chapter according to your truth.

What if minimalism was, in fact, a way of rediscovering the beauty of emptiness? Not an agonising emptiness, but a fertile one. A sacred space, inside and out, where what really matters can finally blossom: inner peace, freedom to be, an authentic connection to yourself and to others.

Because living minimally isn't about living less, it's about living better. With consciously. With heart. With alignment.

As you close this book, don't just take away ideas or methods. Take away an intention. To cultivate simplicity in everything you do. To purify without forcing yourself, to sort without violence, to slow down without feeling guilty. Take with you the certainty that you can, right now, choose a life full of meaning, light and lightness.

Minimalism is a path. Go at your own pace. Every step counts. And remember: you don't need more. You just need something better.

Appendix

Glossary :

A

Hoarding

The tendency to pile up objects, often without any real use, out of habit or fear of running out.

fear of running out. Minimalism encourages us to free ourselves from this tendency.

Minimalist diary

Organising your time by eliminating superfluous commitments and keeping only

those activities that are in line with your priorities.

Self-discipline

The ability to set limits and make conscious choices on a daily basis, even in the absence of an immediate reward.

in the absence of immediate reward. Useful in a minimalist approach.

B

Real need

Genuine need, as opposed to a desire or need artificially created by advertising or

social pressure.

Inner well-being

A feeling of peace and satisfaction resulting from a lifestyle aligned with one's deepest

values, often reinforced by minimalism.

C

Mental burden

The psychological weight of the many tasks to be managed, often invisible. Minimalism helps to lighten this load by simplifying routines.

Mental clarity

A state of lucidity and inner calm encouraged by a pared down environment and clear priorities.

Conscious consumption

Buying less but better, taking into account utility, sustainability and ecological or ethical impact.

Responsible consumption

Choosing to consume in a way that respects resources, people and our own equilibrium.

Unleashed creativity

The ability to create that is reborn when we free ourselves from an overload of objects, information or distractions.

D

Decluttering

The act of sorting, discarding, donating or recycling unnecessary objects to create a clear and functional environment.

Detachment

The ability to free oneself emotionally from material possessions or attachments.

Digital minimalism

Intentional reduction in the use of screens, notifications and social networks
to make better use of time and preserve mental health. E

Inner ecology

Harmonising our inner space (mental, emotional) with our physical space through
simplicity and reducing the superfluous.

Essential

What has lasting and significant value in one's life. The heart of minimalism is to
identify it and devote oneself to it.

Minimalist aesthetic

A refined, sober and functional style that aims for simplicity and harmony in shapes,
colours and objects.

shapes, colours and objects. F

Frugality

A simple, economical lifestyle based on choice rather than deprivation.

FOMO (Fear Of Missing Out)

Fear of missing out on something. Minimalism helps cultivate the opposite:
JOMO.

G

Capsule wardrobe

Limited collection of interchangeable and versatile clothes. Fewer clothes, more style and less daily stress. H

Conscious habits

Routines chosen with intention, aligned with your values and goals. I

Intentionality

Doing things with a clear, well-thought-out purpose. Living intentionally means getting off automatic pilot.

Sober inspiration

The ability to be inspired by the beauty of simplicity and authenticity.

J

JOMO (Joy Of Missing Out)

The pleasure of not doing or following everything. Appreciation of the present moment, even when things are not hectic.

L

Material liberation

The feeling of freedom that comes from letting go of unnecessary possessions.

Less is more

"Less is more": a fundamental principle of minimalism, which values quality over quantity.

quality over quantity. M

Materialism

Value system centred on possession and consumption. Minimalism is a

response to this logic.

Minimalism

The art of living with less in order to concentrate on what really matters.

Emotional minimalism

The practice of not burdening ourselves with toxic emotions, unnecessary conflicts or superficial relationships.

O

Intentional object

An object that has a clear purpose or deep meaning. In a minimalist

In a minimalist interior, everything has a purpose.

P

Full awareness

Paying attention to the present moment, without judgement. It allows you to slow down and savour small pleasures more fully.

Priorities

The most important things in a person's life. Minimalism

is to identify them and devote your time and energy to them.

R

Slow down

Choosing to do things more slowly, consciously, rather than constantly running.

Essential routines

Simple, stable daily activities that provide structure, well-being and mental clarity.

S

Voluntary simplicity

A deliberate choice to live with less, in a quest for meaning, freedom and well-being.

Slow living

A lifestyle that emphasises quality of life, slowness and respect for one's own rhythm.

Sobriety

The art of living in moderation, with simplicity, without excess or

deprivation. T

Free time

Time that is freed up once unnecessary distractions, objects and obligations have been eliminated. It can be used to create, rest or reconnect with oneself.

Overflow

An overload of objects, commitments and thoughts. Minimalism helps to to make room for what's essential.

V

Values

Fundamental principles that guide a minimalist lifestyle. They may include
freedom, authenticity, inner peace or human connection.

Simple living

A life refocused on what is meaningful, free from complications and the race to possess.

The power of emptiness... for a meaningful life

This book was not simply a method of tidying up or a guide to more sober consumption. It was a path. A return to the essentials. An invitation to make room around you and within you for what really matters.

In each chapter, you've explored much more than a lifestyle: a veritable philosophy, an intentional art of living that frees the mind, lightens the heart and gives new depth to every moment.

If you're reading this, you're ready. Ready to declutter, simplify and slow down. But above all, ready to choose: to choose clarity over confusion, quality over quantity, alignment over dispersion.

Minimalism doesn't end here. It starts now. In your daily choices. In your fresh look at your space, your relationships, your time. In every object you let go and every breath you take.

Remember: it's not what you own that defines you, but the space you create to live
to live fully.

Thank you for walking with me. May this book be the start of a simpler... and infinitely richer life.

Claire Montel

Printed in Dunstable, United Kingdom

68264003R00097